Acute Coronary Syndromes

Richard Katz MD, FACC
Professor of Medicine, Director of Division of Cardiology
The George Washington University School of Medicine, Washington DC, USA

Henry Purcell MB, PhD
Senior Fellow in Cardiology
Royal Brompton Hospital, London, UK

Foreword by
Kim Fox MD, FRCP, FESC
President Elect, European Society of Cardiology
Professor of Clinical Cardiology
Imperial College of Science, Technology and Medicine, London, UK
Consultant Cardiologist and Director of Cardiology
Royal Brompton Hospital, London, UK

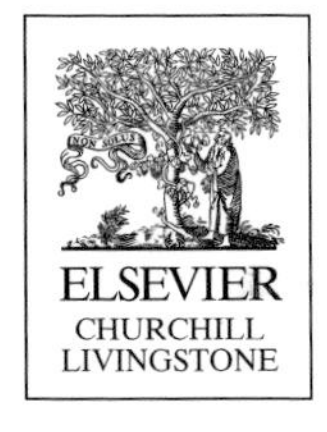

EDINBURGH LONDON NEW YORK OXFORD PHILADELPHIA ST

ELSEVIER
CHURCHILL
LIVINGSTONE

First published 2006
Reprinted 2006

ISBN 0 443 10296 1

British Library Cataloguing in Publication Data
A catalogue record for this book is available from the British Library

Library of Congress Cataloguing in Publication Data
A catalogue record for this book is available from the Library of Congress

Printed in China

Contents

Foreword

Acute coronary syndromes (ACS) remain a major health burden responsible for considerable morbidity and mortality, and the cause of a large number of hospital admissions. Findings from the Euro Heart Survey of ACS and large international registries such as the Global Registry of Acute Coronary Events (GRACE), highlight the unfavourable prognosis of these patients. Recent clinical trials, however, indicate that clinical strategies incorporating careful risk stratification combined with optimal medical therapy, and revascularization in appropriately selected patients, can improve both immediate and long-term clinical outcomes. There is now clear evidence that coronary heart disease mortality rates are falling rapidly in many countries and that there is a declining prevalence of ST elevation myocardial infarction in patients presenting with ACS. Such patterns are likely to reflect improvements in coronary care and in secondary prevention, with better control of conventional cardiovascular risk factors, but much still remains to be done.

This book is therefore timely as it provides a compact but comprehensive overview of the spectrum of ACS. It looks at present and future biomarkers, and methodologies for early risk assessment and diagnosis, as well as the treatments in current use and in the pipeline. Many new drugs are designed to address the underlying pathophysiology, to prevent vulnerable plaque rupture and thrombus formation. I feel that this book will be a valuable contribution and "hands-on" aid to the treatment and prevention of ACS generally, and would recommend it to any doctor who is likely to deal with acute cardiology.

Kim Fox
President Elect, European Society of Cardiology
Professor of Clinical Cardiology
Imperial College of Science, Technology and Medicine, London, UK
Consultant Cardiologist and Director of Cardiology,
Royal Brompton Hospital, London, UK

Acknowledgement

Dedicated to our ever-patient families, and also to Alison Taylor at Elsevier and our own, indefatigable editor, Ann Stringer – with grateful thanks.

Preface

Despite reduced deaths from cardiovascular disease in developed countries acute coronary syndromes (ACS) remain one the most common causes of morbidity and mortality. The presenting features of patients with ACS appear to be changing from a predominance of ST segment elevation myocardial infarction (STEMI) to a scenario where ST elevation is typically absent. The precise reasons for this change are not yet clear but as a recent editorial suggests "the management of patients with acute coronary syndromes may be about to undergo a dramatic change".[1]

In recent years there have been an avalanche of new treatments and clinical trials that have altered the landscape of the treatment of these conditions. International heart societies have published revised consensus guidelines for the therapy for ACS. These guidelines can be complex and rapidly outdated by new clinical information. The purpose of this monograph is to distil and organize the maze of clinical data on the diagnosis, risk stratification, treatment, and prevention of ACS. We and our contributor colleagues discuss pragmatically how to treat NSTEMI and STEMI, looking at some of the oldest drugs we have, such as aspirin, through to the new thrombin inhibitors, lytics and the like. We cannot possibly hope to explore fashionable views on inflammation, infection, reversing endothelial dysfunction, thrombolysis versus primary angioplasty and so forth in great depth, but we do flag up many of the developments in these fields and present the evidence to support the rapidly evolving guidelines.

This book is intended for all those involved in caring for patients with cardiovascular diseases and ACS in particular. This includes nurses, medical students, pharmacists, paramedical workers, the primary care team, general physicians, and of course, cardiologists. We hope that this summary can be used by healthcare professionals to take maximum advantage of the tremendous advances in ACS.

Richard Katz
Professor of Medicine, Director of Division of Cardiology
The George Washington University School of Medicine, Washington DC, USA

Henry Purcell
Senior Fellow in Cardiology
Royal Brompton Hospital, London, UK

Reference

1. Kleiman NS, White HD. The declining prevalence of ST elevation infarction in patients presenting with acute coronary syndromes. Heart 2005;91:1121–1123.

Contributors

Dr Shaheeda Ahmed
Cardiologist
Sunnybrook and Women's College Health Sciences Centre, Toronto, Canada

Dr Nicholas Curzen
Consultant Cardiologist
Wessex Cardiac Unit, Southampton University Hospitals NHS Trust, UK

Dr Miles Dalby
Consultant Cardiologist
Harefield Hospital, Middlesex, UK

Dr Caroline Daly
Cardiology Specialist Registrar
Royal Brompton Hospital, London, UK

Dr C Michael Gibson
Director
TIMI Data Coordinating Center & Angiographic Core Laboratory, Boston, USA
Associate Chief of Cardiology & Director Academic Affairs
Associate Professor, Harvard Medical School
Beth Israel Deaconess Medical Center, Boston, USA

Dr Sandy Gupta
Consultant Cardiologist
Whipps Cross University Hospital and St Bartholomew's Hospital, London, UK

Dr Rob Hatrick
Cardiology Specialist Registrar
Southampton General Hospital, Southampton, UK

Dr Siân Holiday
Specialist Registrar in Geriatrics
St Richard's Hospital, Chichester, UK

Dr Lars Hvilsted Rasmussen
Associate Professor & Director of Cardiology Services
Aalborg Hospital Heart Centre, Aarhus University Hospital, Aalborg, Denmark

Dr Sam Kaddoura
Consultant Cardiologist
Chelsea and Westminster Hospital and Royal Brompton Hospital, London, UK

Dr Paul Kalra
Consultant Cardiologist
Portsmouth Hospitals NHS Trust, Portsmouth, UK

Professor Mike Kirby
Faculty of Health and Human Sciences
The Hertfordshire Primary Care Research Network, University of Hertfordshire, Hatfield, UK

Dr Velmurugan Kuppuswamy
Research Fellow in Cardiology
Whipps Cross University Hospital, London, UK

Dr Mike Mead
General Practitioner
Forest House Medical Centre, Leicester, UK

Dr David Mulcahy
Consultant Cardiologist
Tallaght Hospital, Dublin, Ireland

Dr Savita Peace
General Practitioner
The Surgery, Letchworth, Herts, UK

Dr Duane S Pinto
Assistant Professor of Medicine
Harvard Medical School
Director, Cardiology Fellowship
Interventional Cardiology Section
Beth Israel Deaconess Medical Center, Boston, USA

Dr Kausik Ray
British Heart Foundation International Fellow
TIMI Study Group, Boston, USA

Dr Eliana Reyes
Clinical Fellow in Nuclear Cardiology
Royal Brompton Hospital, London, UK

Dr Francesco Saia
Consultant Cardiologist
Catheterization Laboratory, Institute of Cardiology
University of Bologna, Bologna, Italy

Dr Nalyaka Sambu
Cardiology Specialist Registrar
Portsmouth Hospitals NHS Trust, Portsmouth, UK

Dr Mary Sheppard
Consultant Cardiac Pathologist
Royal Brompton Hospital, London, UK

Dr Peter Stott
General Practitioner
Tadworth Farm Surgery, Tadworth, Surrey, UK

Dr Han Bin Xiao
Cardiologist
Ealing Hospital NHS Trust, Middlesex, UK

Biographies

Richard Katz MD, FACC was appointed the Director of the Division of Cardiology at the George Washington University in 1997. He has been involved in numerous research studies and has served as the principal investigator for a number of national clinical trials including CAST – Cardiac Arrhythmia Suppression Trial, PEACE – Prospective Evaluation of ACE inhibitors and BEST – Beta-blocker Evaluation of Survival Trial. He has presented his research experiences across the country at numerous conferences including those hosted by the American Heart Association and the American College of Cardiology. In addition, his research findings have been published in over 80 articles and more than 100 abstracts.

Dr Katz has been visiting professor to both the Royal Brompton National Heart and Lung Hospital and the Hammersmith Hospital in London, UK. He is a fellow of the American College of Cardiology and served as their governor of the District of Columbia from 1997 to 2000.

He serves on the board of directors for the Larry King Cardiac Foundation and on the editorial boards of *Cardiology Review* and the *British Journal of Cardiology*. In addition, he is a reviewer for *Circulation* and the *American Journal of Cardiology* and a consultant for the National Institute of Health.

Henry Purcell MB, PhD is Senior Fellow in Cardiology at the Royal Brompton Hospital, London. He lectures widely and has published many peer-reviewed research papers and abstracts. He was a member of the British Cardiac Society Working Group producing guidelines on management of patients with acute coronary syndromes without peristent ECG ST segment elevation (2001). He is co-editor of the *British Journal of Cardiology* and sits on several editorial boards, and has co-edited the text *Specialist Training in Cardiology*, published by Elsevier/Mosby. He is also a reviewer for many international journals in cardiovascular medicine.

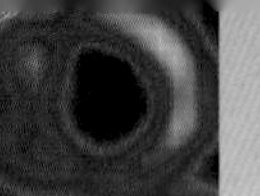

Introduction

Coronary heart disease (CHD) remains the number one cause of death in developed countries, however, the largest projected increases in disease rates are in developing countries. Angina pectoris is the principal manifestation of coronary atherosclerosis. Patients with stable angina are at increased risk of atherosclerotic plaque instability, the development of severe myocardial ischaemia and the development of acute events such as myocardial infarction (MI). In line with the changing patterns of acute events, older descriptions such as sub-endocardial and Q-wave MI have now been replaced with the term acute coronary syndromes (ACS). ACS include unstable angina (UA), non-ST segment elevation myocardial infarction (NSTEMI) and ST-segment elevation myocardial infarction (STEMI).[1]

Acute chest pain is common; in the US more than 6 million patients present to emergency departments with this symptom annually. About 335,000 people a year die of CHD in the emergency room or before reaching hospital. Many patients may initially seek help from their general practitioner, where treatment begins. It then becomes the responsibility of the emergency medicine physician or cardiologist to initiate hospital admission, to continue medical management and to weigh up the need for early coronary intervention. Recent registry data[2] show that hospital admissions are increasing and that UA/NSTEMI is now more common than STEMI.

“Patients with UA or NSTEMI may rapidly progress to STEMI or death within a few hours of symptom onset”

This text reviews the latest thinking in the diagnosis and treatment of ACS. We look at the evidence from clinical trials on which international guidelines and recommendations are based. Our intention is to distil down the vast amount of information on the topic and to provide the reader with pragmatic advice to manage this high-risk patient group. This book is aimed at all healthcare workers, both in hospitals and in primary care as well as medical students who are involved in the care of cardiac patients. We hope that you find it interesting and informative.

General concepts of ACS

Definitions

Variation in prognosis, and treatment, along with the advent of new “biomarkers” and advances in imaging techniques, led to a joint European Society of Cardiology (ESC)/American College of Cardiology (ACC) redefinition of MI in the context of ACS.[3] ACS patients are divided into those *without* and those *with* ST-segment elevation. The ACS *without* ST elevation include both UA and NSTEMI (Figure 1). UA is further defined as ischaemic pain at rest without elevation of biomarkers, whereas NSTEMI requires increased

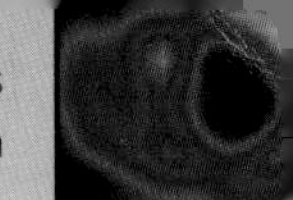

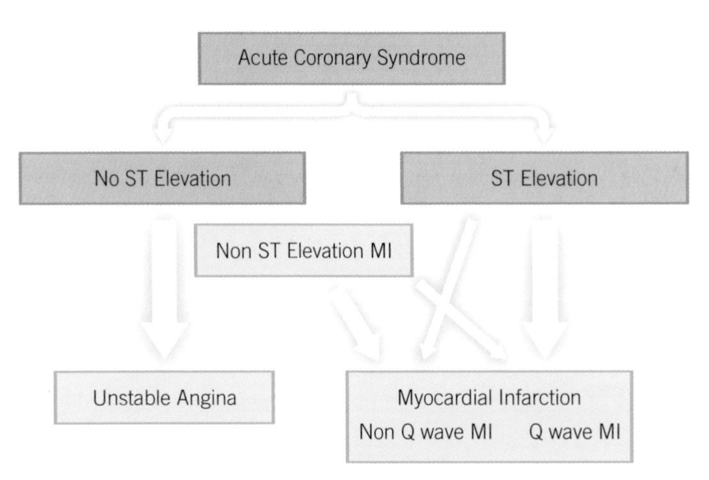

Fig. 1 Nomenclature of ACS. Reproduced with permission from Committee on the Management of Patients with Unstable Angina. ACC/AHA Guidelines for the Management of Patients with Unstable Angina and Non-ST-Segment Elevation Myocardial Infarction. *J Am Coll Cardiol* 2000;36:970–1062. © Elsevier

serum biomarkers. STEMI has both ST-segment and biomarker elevation. Using these criteria, MI (either NSTEMI or STEMI) is defined as myocardial cell death due to prolonged ischaemia irrespective of electrocardiogram (ECG) changes. Myocardial necrosis can be confirmed by the appearance of different proteins (biomarkers) released into the circulation by damaged myocytes. These include myoglobin (MB), cardiac troponins T (TnT) and I (TnI), creatinine kinase myoglobin (CK-MB) and total creatinine kinase (CK). The timing of release of these biomarkers after MI is shown in Figure 2.[4]

Epidemiology

This year an estimated 700,000 Americans will have a "new coronary attack" and about 500,000 will have a recurrent attack.[5] Heart disease is predominantly a disease of the elderly (Figure 3). The first event occurs at an average age of 65.8 years for men and 70.4 years for women. Some 50% of men and 63% of women who die suddenly from CHD have no previous symptoms of the disease. Studies evaluating the percentage of ACS patients who have STEMI range from 30 to 45%. US figures put a conservative estimate of 928,000 people with ACS discharged from hospital in 2001, however when secondary discharge diagnoses are included the corresponding number of discharges becomes 1,680,000 unique hospitalizations for ACS, 959,000 for MI and 758,000 for UA.

"Older patients and those with ventricular dysfunction fare worst after MI"

Throughout Europe CHD also remains the leading cause of mortality in men and women, accounting for nearly 2 million deaths annually.

It is difficult to estimate the incidence of ACS in the UK and it is thought that there may be variations in the coding of this condition leading to underestimates of the actual rates. Estimates suggest that

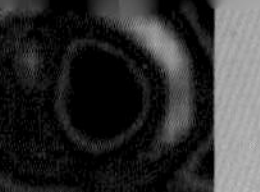

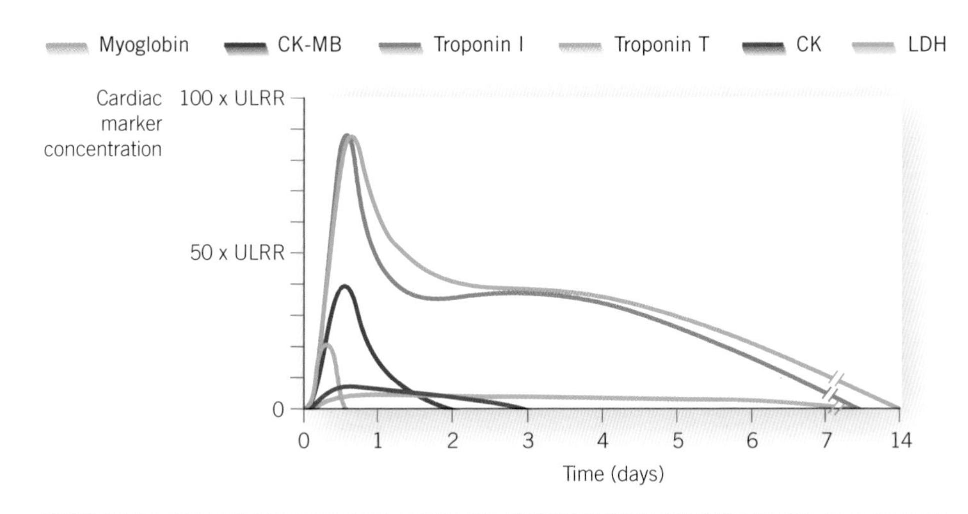

Properties of cardiac marker proteins

Protein	Molecular mass (kD)	First detection*	Duration of detection	Sensitivity	Specificity
Fatty acid binding protein	12	1.5–2 hours	8–12 hours	+++	++
Myoglobin	16	1.5–2 hours	8–12 hours	+++	+
CK-MB	83	2–3 hours	1–2 days	+++	+++
Troponin I	33	3–4 hours	7–10 days	++++	++++
Troponin T	38	3–4 hours	7–14 days	++++	++++
CK	96	4–6 hours	2–3 days	++	++
Aspartate transaminase	~103	6–10 hours	3–5 days	++	+
LDH	135	6–10 hours	5–7 days	++	+

Fig. 2 Timing of biomarker release after MI. LDH = lactate dehydrogenase. Reproduced with permission from French JK, White HD. Clinical implications of the new definition of myocardial infarction. *Heart* 2004;90:99–106. © BMJ Publishing Group

there are approximately 120,000 new cases of ACS per annum in England and Wales. Recent data from Scotland[6] suggest that, while the incidence of acute MI decreased (by about 33%) between 1990 and 2000, hospitalization rates for angina increased by 79%, for chest pain by 110%, and for any suspected ACS (MI, angina or chest pain) by 25% (Figure 4).

The reason for this decline in acute MI and the shift towards presentation with ACS is unexplained. It may be related to:

- enhanced risk assessment and improved diagnosis (e.g. new biomarkers) with better coding and classification for hospital discharge statistics
- new evidence-based treatment regimens and widespread use of aspirin.

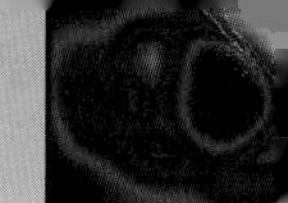

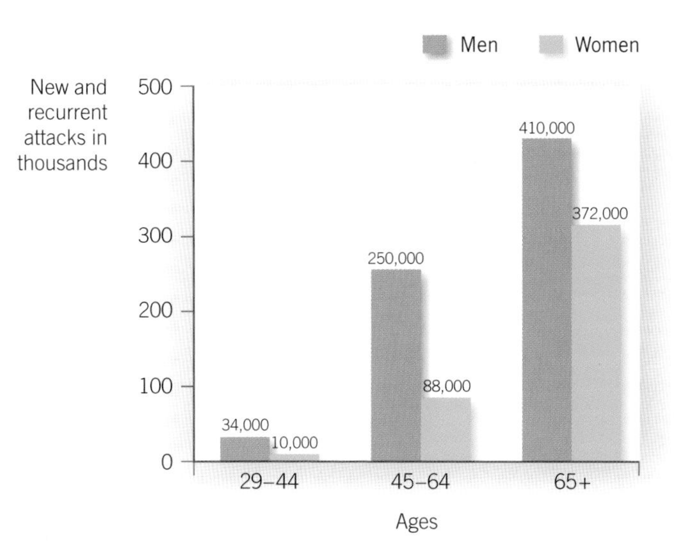

Fig. 3 Annual number of Americans having coronary attacks.
Reproduced with permission from American Heart Association. Heart Disease and Stroke Statistics – 2005 Update. © American Heart Association.

Prognosis

Earlier information from the Duke University Medical Center Database showed that risk of adverse outcome in acute ischaemia is especially high soon after the onset of symptoms and declines relatively quickly, approaching that of stable coronary disease after 2–3 months (Figure 5).[7] Findings from two large International surveys, GRACE[2] and Euro Heart Survey ACS,[8] involving over 22,000 ACS patients show increasing event rates with increasing disease severity. These observations are borne out in a study conducted in east London in 1225 patients with acute MI.[9] This showed that 30% of acute MI patients and 20% with UA experience a major event (death or non-fatal coronary syndrome) during the first year after hospital admission. Some 66% of all major events during the first 6 months post-MI occur in the first 30 days. For hospitalized patients survival is determined importantly by advanced age and presence of ventricular dysfunction (Figure 6), with residual myocardial ischaemia and cardiac arrhythmias contributing significantly.[10] More recent long-term findings from GRACE[11] also show continuing poor outcomes for ACS patients (Figure 7), with around one in five patients requiring hospitalization for heart disease during the 6 months' follow-up, and approximately 15% undergoing revascularization.

"These complications highlight the importance of an aggressive early treatment strategy for UA/NSTEMI similar to STEMI patients"

These data underline the need for better long-term medical management of ACS patients.

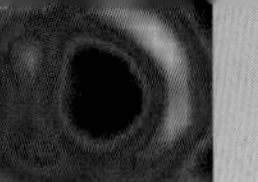

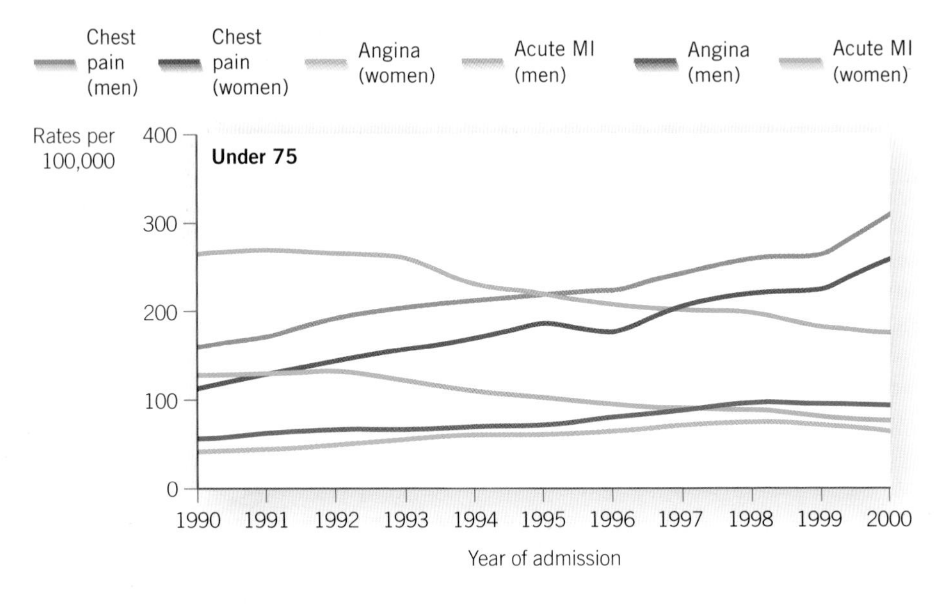

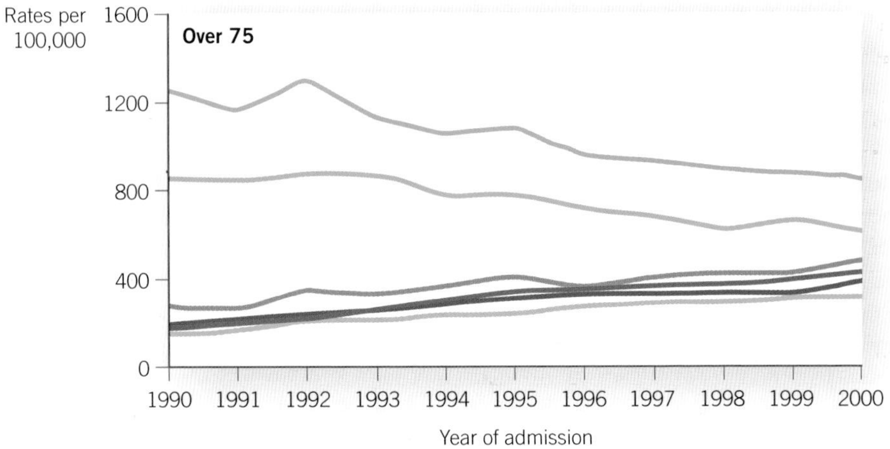

Fig. 4 Hospital discharge rates for suspected ACS between 1990 and 2000: population-based analysis.

Reproduced with permission from Murphy NF, MacIntyre K, Capewell S, et al. Hospital discharge rates for suspected acute coronary syndromes between 1990 and 2000: population based analysis. *BMJ* 2004;328:1413–1414. © BMJ Publishing Group

Pathophysiology

UA, NSTEMI and STEMI are closely related conditions with similar pathogenesis and clinical presentation, but with differing severity. They differ primarily in whether the ischaemia is severe enough to cause sufficient myocardial damage to release detectable levels of indicators of myocardial injury, such as troponins.

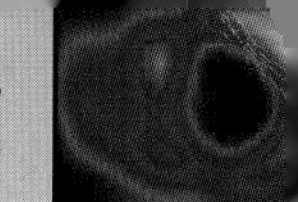

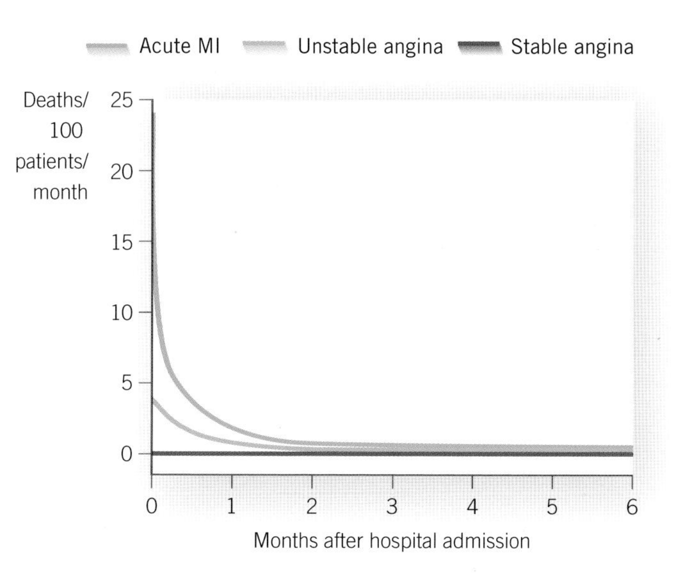

Fig. 5 Adverse outcome in acute ischaemia over time. Outcome of 21,761 patients with ACS. Reproduced from Agency for Health Care Policy and Research, National Heart, Lung and Blood Institute: Unstable angina: diagnosis and management, clinical practice guideline no. 10. Rockville, MD, US Department of Health and Human Services, Public Health Service, AHCPR Publication no. 94-0602, March 1994.

The pathophysiology of atherosclerosis and ACS is well characterized. The earliest visible atherosclerotic lesion appears to be the fatty streak (Figure 8). Beginning in early life, these fatty streaks, or Type II lesions, are slightly raised above the intimal surface and predominantly contain foam cells derived from tissue macrophages and T lymphocytes. Many of these fatty streaks progress to become advanced atherosclerotic plaques. The earliest detectable *physiological* manifestation of atherosclerosis is reduced production of the endothelium-dependent vasodilator, nitric oxide (NO).[12] NO is synthesized from the amino acid L-arginine by means of the enzyme NO synthase (e-NOS), and it is released from endothelial cells in response to shear stress from blood flow and the activation of a variety of receptors. NO also has important anti-inflammatory, antithrombogenic and antiproliferative properties. Endothelial function can be assessed in a number of ways, notably with forearm strain gauge plethysmography or high-resolution ultrasound to measure changes in flow-mediated endothelium-dependent dilatation (FMD) following the infusion of endothelium-dependent vasodilators such as acetylcholine.

"Endothelial dysfunction and its associated reduced synthesis of NO predisposes to atherosclerosis"

Endothelial dysfunction is characterized by a reduction of the bioavailability of vasodilators such as NO, and an increase in endothelium-derived contracting factors, including endothelin and angiotensin II (AII). The imbalance between these "good guys and bad guys" results in endothelial dysfunction, sometimes referred to as "the Risk of the Risk Factors" (Figure 9).[12] Endothelial dysfunction predisposes to atherogenesis and is a marker of atherosclerotic risk. A number

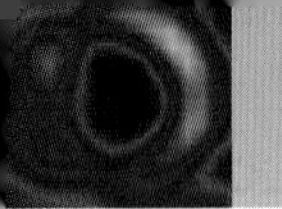

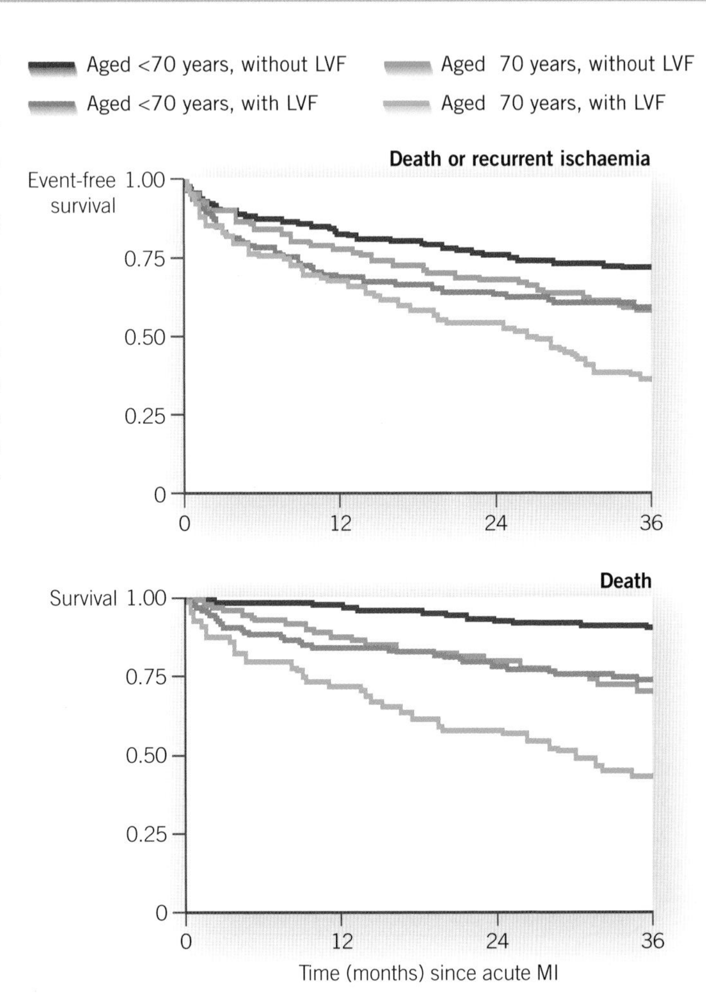

Fig. 6 Kaplan-Meier curves. Overall and event-free survival by age for patients surviving to hospital discharge. LVF = left ventricular failure. Reproduced with permission from Barakat K, Wilkinson P, Deaner A, et al. How should age affect management of acute myocardial infarction? A prospective cohort study. *Lancet* 1999;353:955–959. © Elsevier

of drugs that have been shown to reduce cardiovascular events, such as angiotensin converting enzyme (ACE) inhibitors and statins, also improve (reverse) endothelial dysfunction. Endothelial dysfunction appears to play a fundamental role in the development of ACS.

“Endothelial vasodilator dysfunction may serve as a marker of vascular risk”

Fatty streaks may progress to become mature plaques (Figure 10).[13,14] Platelets adhere to the initial lesion and secrete growth factors including platelet-derived growth factor (PDGF) that initiate smooth muscle cell migration from the media to the intima. This in turn stimulates the production of collagen, elastin and glycoproteins, which provide the connective tissue matrix of the plaque and give it structural strength. Extracellular cholesterol, derived from low-density lipoprotein (LDL)-cholesterol or from decaying lipid-containing macrophage foam cells, begins to accumulate within the matrix

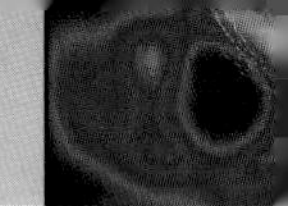

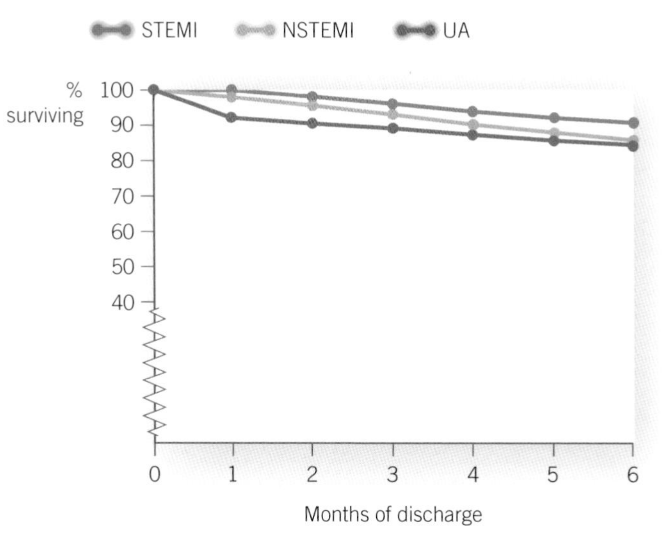

Fig. 7 Poor outcomes in GRACE. Reproduced with permission from Goldberg RJ, Currie K, White K, et al. The Global Registry of Acute Coronary Events GRACE. *Am J Cardiol* 2004;93:288–293. © Elsevier

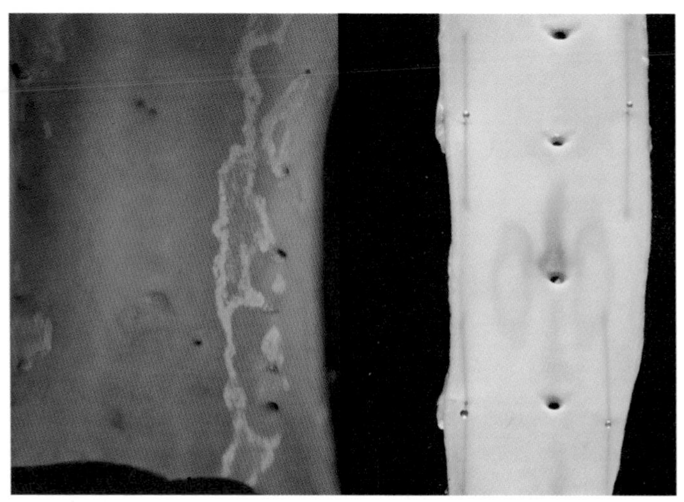

Fig. 8 Fatty streak. Far left shows aorta opened to reveal fatty streaks on the intimal surface. Far right shows fatty streak stained red, indicating fat deposition in the intima near branching point. Young adult aged 15.

forming a lipid core within the lesion, which becomes more elevated. The lesion then becomes covered by a fibromuscular cap consisting of smooth muscle cells and collagen with a single layer of endothelial cells. This whole entity is referred to as a raised fibrolipid or advanced plaque, and becomes the substrate for plaque complications and the development of clinical symptoms.

Some plaques may cause severe stenoses while many remain angiographically invisible and begin to bulge into the adventitia rather than towards the lumen, a process referred to as Glagovian remodelling (Figure 11). This is where the arterial media remodels to allow the

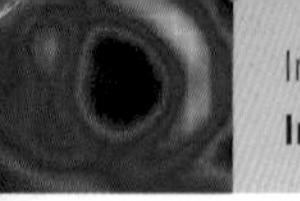

Local factors
Non-traditional risk factors
Traditional risk factors
Genetic predisposition
Unknown factors

Endothelial Dysfunction: "the Risk of the Risk Factors"

Vascular lesion and remodelling
Inflammation
Vasoconstriction
Thrombosis
Plaque rupture/erosion

Fig. 9 Endothelial dysfunction – risk of risk factors. Reproduced with permission from Bonetti PO, Lerman LO, Lerman A. Endothelial dysfunction. A marker of atherosclerotic risk. Arterioscler Thromb Vasc Biol 2003;23:168–175. © Lippincott Williams & Wilkins

vessel to increase its cross sectional area and thereby accommodate the plaque without any reduction in luminal area (compensatory dilatation).

Cholesterol is constantly transported in and out of atheroscerotic plaques. It enters in the form of LDL and lipoprotein (a) – Lp(a). Plaque lipid content decreases after a reduction in serum cholesterol levels in animal models, and there continues to be much interest in the use of drugs that may modify the composition of these lesions to cause stabilization and bring about a "quiescent coronary plaque".[13]

Plaque rupture

The rupture of an atherosclerotic plaque can initiate a range of complications from UA and acute MI through to sudden cardiac

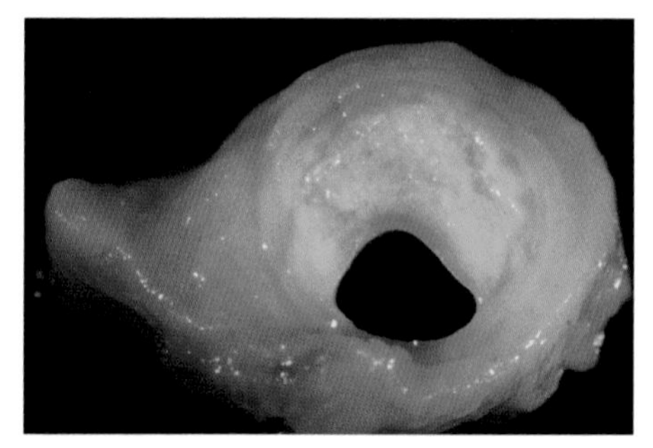

Fig. 10 Mature plaque. With dense fibrins and little lipid involving 50% of circumference of the coronary vessel.

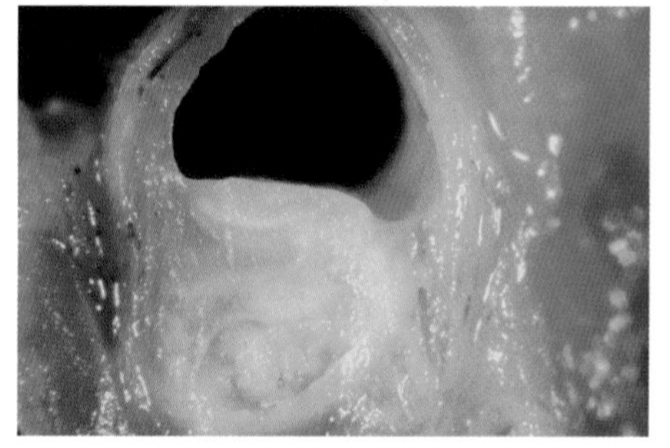

Fig. 11 Glagovian remodelling. Large plaque in coronary artery. Note lumen is not compromised because the plaque has remodelled out into the adventitia of the vessel.

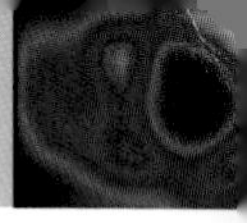

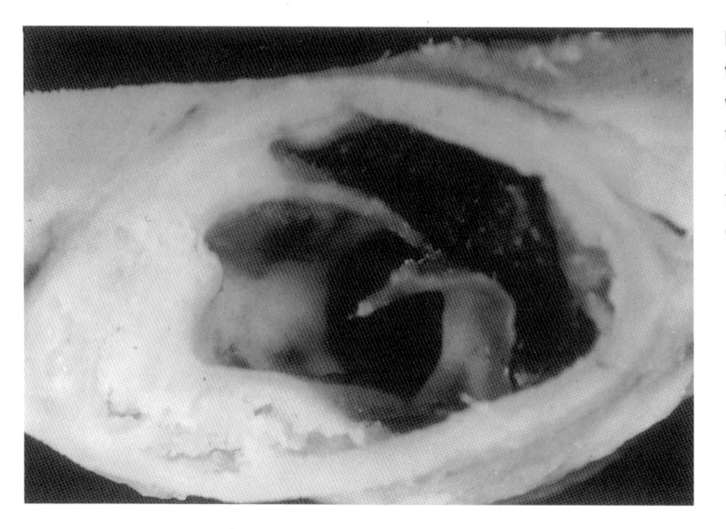

Fig. 12 Plaque cap tear. Vulnerable plaque with large lipid core and thin cap that has ruptured with release of thrombogenic lipid contents.

death. Such disruption is common and often clinically silent with about 10% of "normal" individuals having asymptomatic disrupted plaques in their coronary arteries. The clinical presentation and outcome depend on the location, severity and duration of myocardial ischaemia.

Acute coronary occlusion usually occurs through one of two distinct processes.[14] First, the endothelium covering the atherosclerotic plaque can become denuded (endothelial erosion) with exposure of the prothrombotic subendothelium to the circulating blood. Second, plaque disruption may occur with the tearing open of the fibrous cap (plaque rupture) to expose the highly thrombogenic lipid core. Plaque disruption may range from minor (superficial) to major (deep) fissures leading to differing intensity platelet-fibrin accumulation (Figure 12). The type of thrombus (platelet plug or platelet-fibrin thrombus) and the extent and duration of obstruction to coronary blood flow determine the effect on the myocardium with the development of UA, NSTEMI, or STEMI. Figure 13 shows the anatomical changes from the vulnerable plaque leading to the process of disruption and ACS and remodelling.[15]

"Rupture or endothelial erosion of a plaque with subsequent thrombosis represents the substrate of ACS"

Plaque rupture depends more on the type of plaque than its size. Major determinants of plaque vulnerability include both local and systemic factors (Figure 14).[16] Local factors include size and consistency of the atheromatous core, thickness of the fibrous cap, ongoing inflammation and repair within the cap, eccentric (as distinct from concentric) plaque shape, and shear forces. The shear forces include coronary tone and pressure, bending and twisting of the artery with cardiac contractility and coronary spasm. Systemic factors

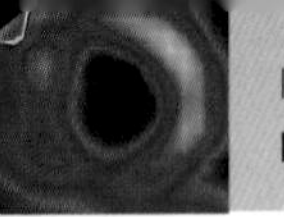

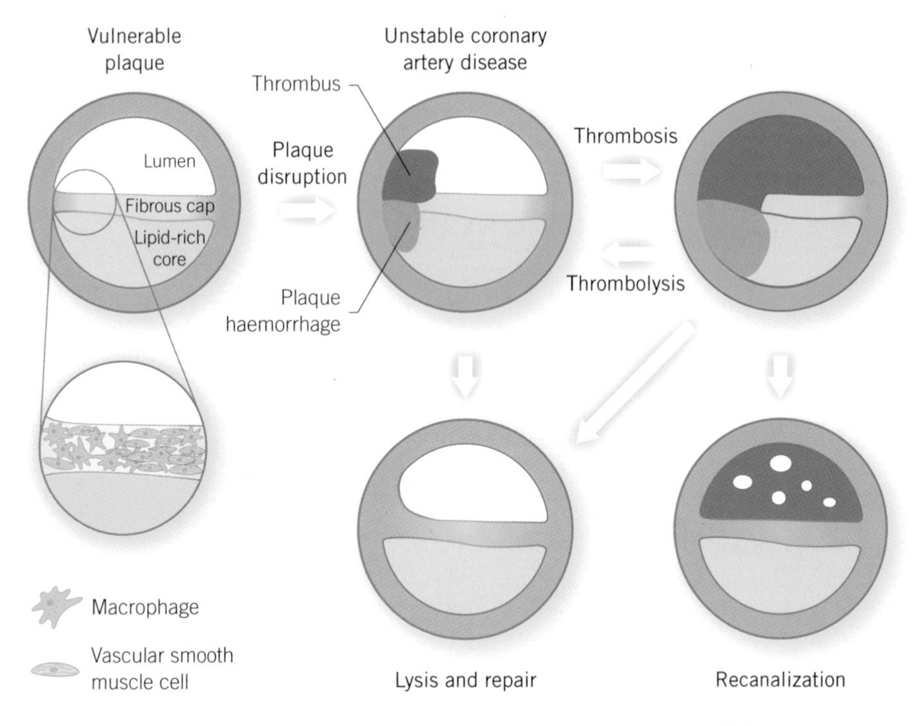

Fig. 13 Plaque disruption and remodelling. Reproduced with permission from Theroux P, Fuster V. Acute coronary syndromes. Unstable angina and non-Q-wave myocardial infarction. Circulation 1998;97:1195–1206. © Lippincott Williams & Wilkins

promoting plaque rupture include physical "triggers" (e.g. exertion in normally sedentary individuals), and high levels of psychological stress[17] with attendant increased adrenergic tone, shear forces, and generalized inflammation.

The milieu of the plaque is also fundamental to its vulnerability. Several lines of evidence have implicated matrix metalloproteinases (MMPs) as major players in plaque rupture. MMPs are a complex group of proteinases with important roles in cardiovascular physiology and pathology.[18] Their ability to degrade fibrous caps makes them an important target for future drug development for the prevention of ACS. Other therapeutic targets are clear from the observation that substantial quantities of AII are also present in atherosclerotic lesions. AII may contribute to vascular dysfunction in atherosclerosis not only through stimulation of smooth muscle cell proliferation but also by increasing cholesterol accumulation and foam cell formation. LDL cholesterol, particularly if oxidized, may be one of the important triggers of inflammation.[19]

Inflammation

"Atherosclerosis is clearly an inflammatory disease and does not result simply from the accumulation of lipids" as outlined by Russell Ross in

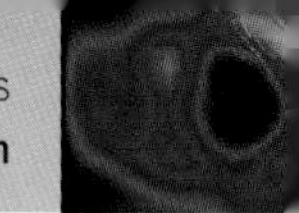

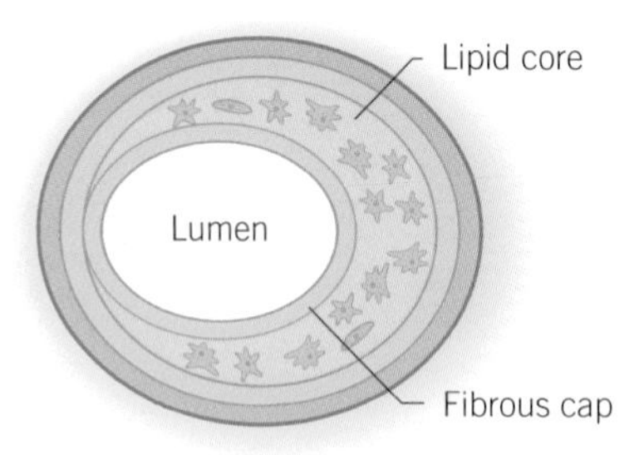

Vulnerable plaque
- Thin fibrous cap
- Inflammatory cell infiltrates: proteolytic activity
- Lipid-rich plaque

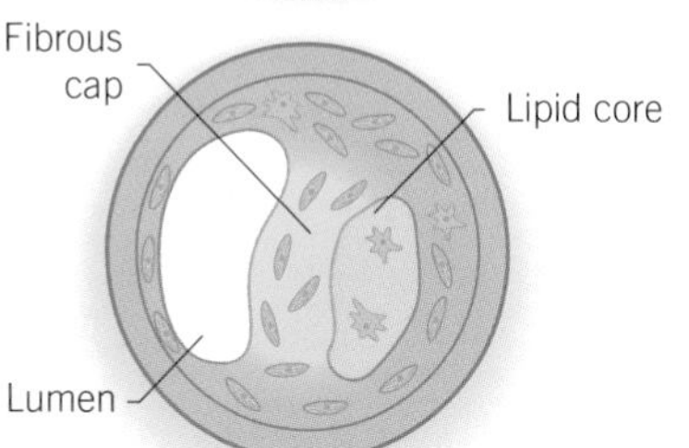

Stable plaque
- Thick fibrous cap
- Smooth muscle cells: more extracellular matrix
- Lipid-poor plaque

Fig. 14 Determinants of plaque vulnerability.

a keynote review article in 1999.[20] This concept has been extended further in a highly recommended recent review by Hansson.[21] Recent studies suggest that coronary instability in ACS is not solely due to a single vulnerable plaque, but that low grade coronary inflammation is widespread throughout the coronary tree.[22] Inflammation is mediated by oxidized lipids as described above and also by reactive oxygen species, inflammatory cytokines, AII, diabetes, infection (Chlamydial heat shock protein), and activation of the immune system, which can destabilize lesions. Much has been published on the putative role of chronic infection involving agents such as *Chlamydia pneumoniae*, cytomegalovirus and so forth as triggers or promoters of inflammation and atherosclerosis. Myocardial virus persistence has been shown to be associated with endothelial dysfunction. High virus titres would therefore appear to be further likely targets for antibiotic treatment, trials to date have however been disappointing (see pages 122–126).

“Elevated levels of inflammatory markers like CRP suggest that local inflammatory mechanisms may contribute to plaque instability”

The factors described above recruit inflammatory cells into the atherosclerotic lesion by increasing the production of adhesion molecules (ICAM, VCAM), chemotactic proteins (monocyte chemoattractant protein-1), interleukins, and C-reactive protein (CRP). Some of the host of current inflammatory mediators and markers implicated in atherogenesis are shown in Figure 15.[19]

CRP, an acute phase reactant produced in the liver in response to interleukin-6 (Il-6), is both a marker and mediator of vascular inflammation as well as being a predictor of coronary events in patients with stable and unstable angina.[23] Inflammation predisposes to fibrous

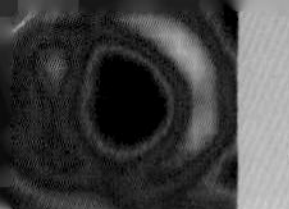

Fig. 15 Inflammatory mediators and markers implicated in atherogenesis. Reproduced from Schachter M. Lipid lowering drugs, inflammation and cardiovascular disease. Br J Diabetes Vasc Dis 2003;3:178–182.

Acute phase proteins (possible markers as well as mediators)
C-reactive protein Fibrinogen Serum amyloid A
Cytokines (modulators of inflammation, both pro- and anti-inflammatory)
Interleukin-6 Interleukin-8 Tumour necrosis factor-α Monocyte chemoattractant protein–1 Interferon-γ
Adhesion molecules (involved in the interaction of endothelial and inflammatory cells)
ICAM-1 VCAM-1 P-selectin E-selectin
Transcription factor (coordination of many genes involved in the inflammatory response)
Nuclear factor-κB

cap rupture by activating MMPs and promoting chronic injury to the vascular endothelium. Arterial endothelial integrity is critical in preserving vascular haemostasis. Endothelial dysfunction results in a pro-thrombotic environment and enhances pro-inflammatory signalling.

Traditional assays for CRP do not have adequate sensitivity for vascular disease prediction, however high-sensitivity CRP (hsCRP) assays have been developed and are now widely available. Levels of CRP and Il-6 are elevated in patients with UA and MI: high levels predict worse prognosis. A moderately elevated hsCRP, even in a healthy population, is an independent risk factor for CHD, but it is still debatable whether this test should be used to screen asymptomatic individuals. The cost of CRP screening is comparable with that of standard cholesterol, and it can be highly cost-effective when combined with LDL-cholesterol results. Ridker considers that the most forseeable use for CRP testing in the emergency room setting will be among those with chest pain syndromes who have negative troponin levels.[24] Patients with negative troponins and negative CRP levels in this setting "are unlikely to have flow limiting coronary disease", he suggests. Levels of CRP used to determine risk are discussed below.

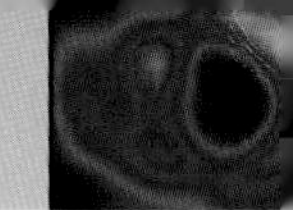

While optimal risk stratification is of paramount importance in ACS, the quest for "new markers" will continue apace. One of the latest such markers, N-Terminal pro-Brain Natriuretic Peptide (NT-proBNP), appears promising in this respect.[25] Experimental evidence also suggests a potential role for serum homocysteine as a predictor of long-term survival in patients with ACS, and further investigational work is ongoing.

"Platelet activation may occur in response to a wide number of stimuli and is key to formation of thrombi"

Platelets and the coagulation system

Platelet activation is an essential step in the formation of platelet-rich thrombi: platelets must be activated for aggregation to occur. Platelet activation is triggered by a wide variety of biochemical and mechanical stimuli. These platelet agonists include adenosine diphospate (ADP), adrenaline, collagen (present following plaque rupture), and thromboxane (released by activated platelets and thrombin – a product of the coagulation cascade).[26] When platelets are activated they undergo morphological and functional changes. When quiescent, in the resting state, platelets have a flat discoid appearance (Figure 16a) but on activation, in this case following exposure to ADP, they become more spherical and adopt pseudopod extensions (Figure 16b). These interact with the extensions of other platelets (Figure 16c) to form platelet thrombi. This platelet aggregation results from the activation of membrane glycoprotein (GP) IIb/IIIa receptors, which in turn bind with fibrinogen molecules, the molecular "glue" of thrombi, and the GP IIb/IIIa receptors of other platelets (Figure 17). The GP IIb/IIIa receptor is responsible for platelet aggregation and is regarded as the final common pathway for platelet-platelet interaction (see pages 59–62).

"The GP IIb/IIIa receptor is responsible for platelet aggregation and is the final common pathway for platelet-platelet interaction"

Following plaque rupture, exposure either of the subendothelium or the lipid core releases tissue factor and other prothrombotic substances into the circulating blood. These factors promote localized platelet adhesion, activation and aggregation. Platelet activation causes degranulation with release of adhesive proteins, prothrombotic factors, pro-inflammatory factors and platelet agonists, which amplify and sustain the acute atherothombotic process. Tissue factor also stimulates the coagulation cascade to produce thrombin, which further amplifies platelet activation and directly promotes fibrin formation. Initially, platelet aggregation results in formation of an intraluminal "platelet plug" with partial or total vessel obstruction.

UA is typified by brief total or near total coronary stenosis with transient rest pain and ST depression on the ECG. Since ischaemic time is short and there is no platelet embolization of the microvasculature, serum troponin levels remain in the normal range. In contrast, NSTEMI is typified by partial or transient platelet plug

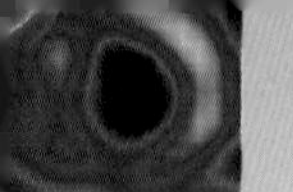

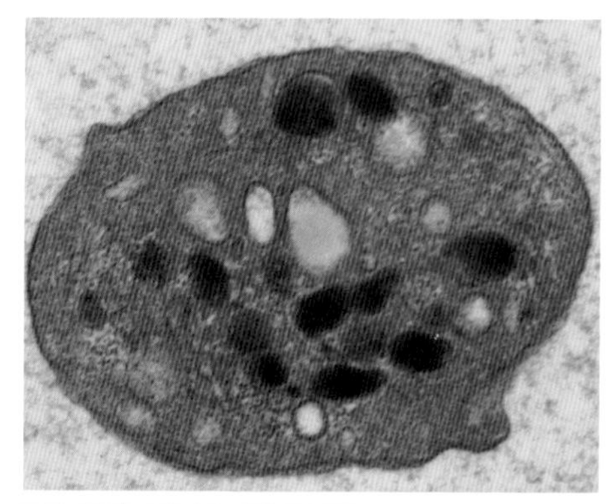

Fig. 16a Quiescent ovoid platelet. Transmission electron micrograph: magnification x 25 000.

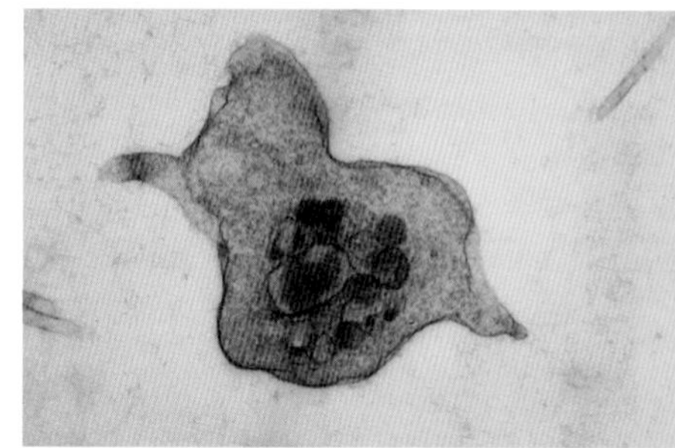

Fig. 16b 10 seconds: note shape change on exposure to ADP, centralization of granules and pseudopod formation. Transmission electron micrograph: magnification x 25 000.

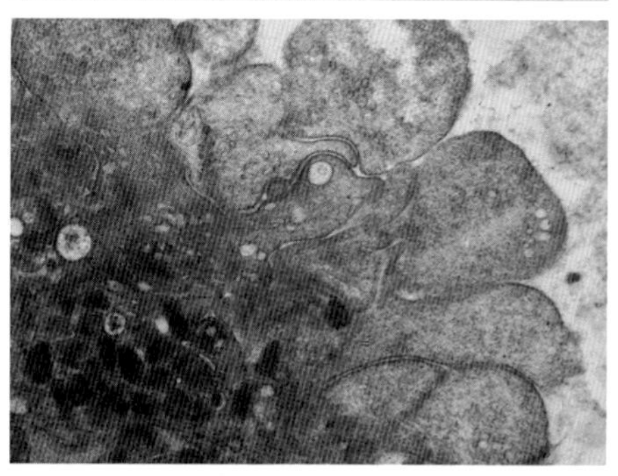

Fig. 16c 4 minutes: note platelet aggregate with interdigitated platelets locked together. Transmission electron micrograph: magnification x 8000.

occlusion of the coronary macrovasculature plus distal embolization of small platelet clumps into the microvasculature. The microemboli result in microscopic MIs, "infarctlets", identified by elevated troponin levels. Since these infarctions can be extremely small there may not be detectable elevation of total CK or CK-MB.

Platelet aggregation and activation of the coagulation cascade can progress from pure platelet mass (plug) to formation of a large platelet-fibrin thrombus. This more "durable" platelet-fibrin thrombus can occlude the coronary macrovasculature with prolonged obstruction producing a large zone of myocardial damage typified by a STEMI and release of all biomarkers/enzymes.

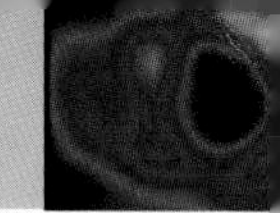

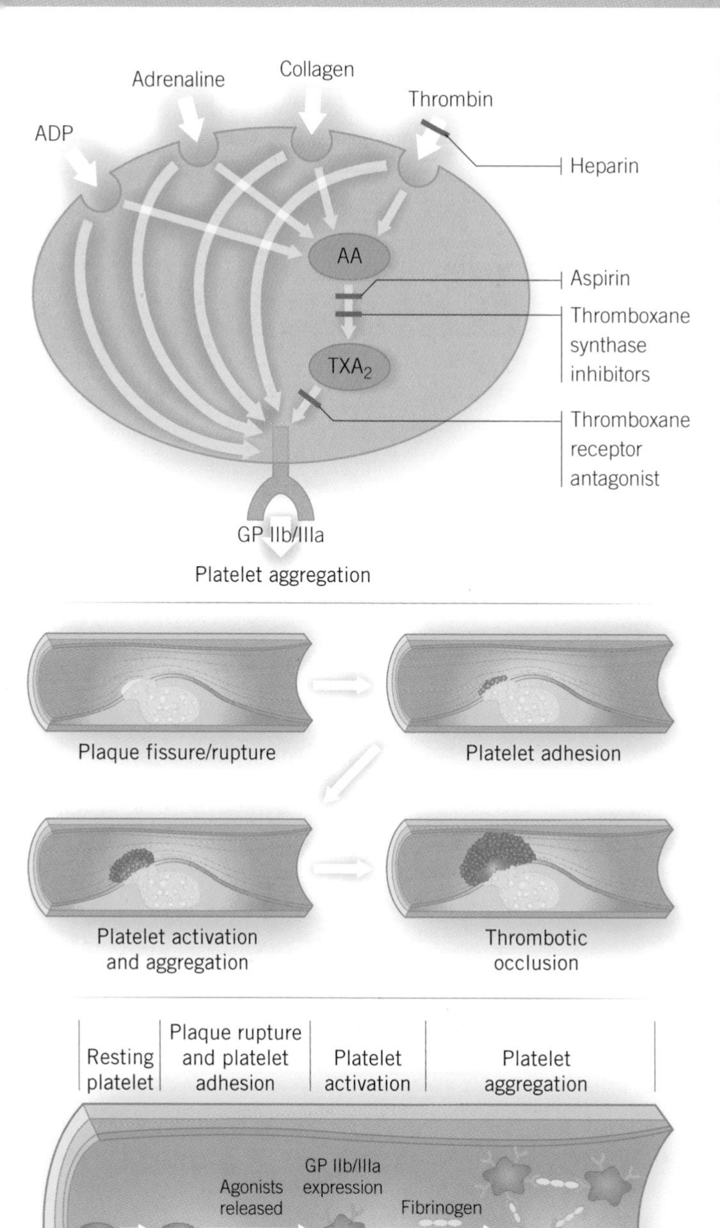

Fig. 17 GP IIb/IIIa – the final common pathway in platelet activation and aggregation.
TXA_2 = thromboxane A_2; AA = arachidonic acid

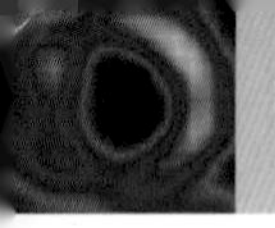

Diagnosis of ACS

“Not all chest pain is cardiac, but consider that it is until proven otherwise”

Over 6 million patients in the US alone present to the emergency department each year with acute chest pain or symptoms suggestive of acute cardiac ischaemia.[27] Over half of them are admitted to rule out ACS. Following hospital admission, approximately 85 to 90% of these patients will be found to have no evidence of ACS. This high proportion of unnecessary hospitalizations is the result of the current limitations in diagnosing acute ischaemic heart disease on presentation. Early diagnosis of ACS is straightforward in the presence of typical symptoms and characteristic ECG features of myocardial ischaemia and necrosis. However, most patients with acute chest pain exhibit a normal or nondiagnostic ECG, which leads to hospital admission for further evaluation. On the other hand, a small but not negligible proportion of patients (5 to 8% in most series) with chest pain and nondiagnostic ECGs are discharged from the emergency department with an evolving acute MI, which often carries a high mortality risk. Therefore, despite the low incidence of ACS in the emergency department and chest pain centres' populations, the threshold for hospital admission remains low because of the high morbidity and mortality risk associated with it. Serum cardiac biomarker analysis has been found to be of great value in the diagnosis of acute myocardial injury; however, its usefulness is limited by a timing factor. Because of their release kinetics, serum biomarkers are only detectable until several hours after the onset of myocardial injury. Moreover, a typical rise and fall pattern of serum levels is required in order for the test to be considered diagnostic. The inability to accurately risk-stratify patients on presentation leads to unnecessary admissions, increased costs and reduction in coronary care bed availability. There is therefore need for a highly specific diagnostic tool that would separate patients with a high probability of ACS from those with a low likelihood who can be discharged home safely. This would expedite the decision-making process leading to better management, quality of care and adequate use of resources.

Patients with chest pain can be categorized into those with:

“All chest pain patients should have a resting 12-lead ECG”

- non-cardiac chest pain
- stable angina
- UA
- NSTEMI or STEMI.

This classification allows risk stratification and selection of an appropriate treatment strategy. Diagnosis is initially based on:

1. Clinical signs and symptoms.
2. Resting 12-lead ECG.
3. Cardiac enzymes/biomarkers.

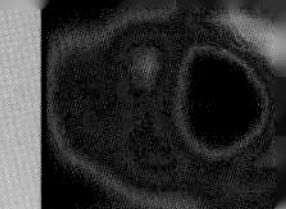

Clinical signs and symptoms

Patients with ACS include those who have experienced any of:

- new onset exertional chest pain typical of ischaemia
- accelerating pattern of previously stable angina (especially at rest or within 2 weeks post-MI)
- ischaemic chest pain at rest.

As recommended clearly in revised guidelines[28] patients with possible ACS should not be evaluated solely over the telephone but "should be referred to a facility that allows evaluation by a physician and the recording of a 12-lead ECG".

Chest pain evaluation

Figure 18 provides an algorithm for the evaluation of acute chest pain from the European Task Force on the management of chest pain.[29] There are important "clues" to pick up on when assessing patients with chest pain. For example, the pain of UA does not usually persist for

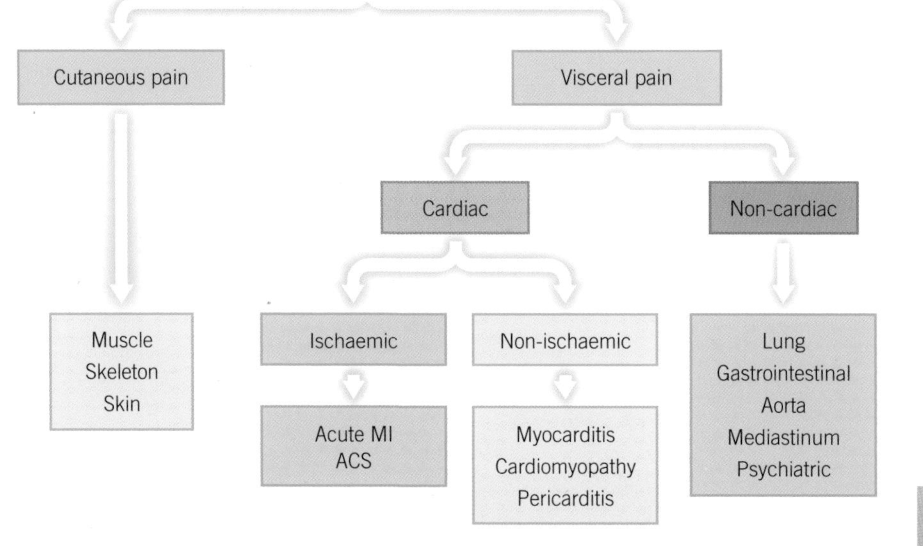

Fig. 18 Algorithm for the diagnosis of acute chest pain. Reproduced with permission from Erhardt L, Herlitz J, Bossaert L, et al. Task force on the management of chest pain. Eur Heart J 2002;23:1153–1176. © Oxford Journals

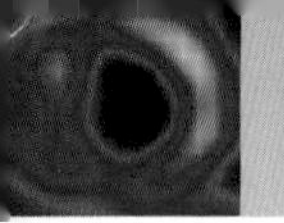

“Outcome is unrelated to symptom severity in ACS”

longer than 20 minutes. Acute MI (either NSTEMI or STEMI) is suspected when pain lasts 20 minutes or more. Chest pain associated with ACS occasionally, but inconsistently, improves with sublingual glyceryl trinitrate (nitroglycerin). Although nitrates may improve the pain, they provide minimal, if any, relief when there is an MI. It should be noted that pain relief after nitrates is *not specific* for ischaemia since nitrates also may improve chest discomfort secondary to oesophageal spasm.

Clues for cardiac pain are a previous history of coronary artery disease (CAD), and radiation of pain to neck, lower jaw or left arm. The pain may not be severe, particularly in the elderly, and other presentations such as fatigue, dyspnoea, faintness or syncope are common. Many patients have evidence of pallor, sweating, and either hypotension or a narrow pulse pressure. Pulse irregularity, bradycardia or tachycardia, a third heart sound and basal rales may also be present.

Clinical history is important for both the diagnosis and risk stratification of patients with ACS. Age, traditional CAD risk factors, use of aspirin, and frequency of rest chest pain episodes are independent risks for adverse outcome. Sudden onset, “knife-like” pain is more likely to have non-ischaemic causes such as oesophageal spasm or to be musculoskeletal, for example. UA is noted at rest or with minimal activity. The pain associated with MI can be described by patients as “terrifying … and intolerable” it tends to be of longer duration (>30 minutes) and is severe and retrosternal.

Outcome is not related to symptom severity in ACS patients. Patients may describe a spectrum from “slight chest discomfort” to “the worst pain I have ever known”. Women may use terms such as “tearing” and “frightening” more frequently than men, who describe the pain as “grinding” for example. The pain may be diffuse over a wide area rather than localized, and it may radiate to the left and/or right arms as well as to the neck, back or jaw. Differential diagnoses of chest pain are outlined in Figure 19.

Differential diagnosis of chest pain

Cardiac causes	Non-cardiac causes
Aortic stenosis	Oesophageal reflux/spasm
Hypertrophic cardiomyopathy	Peptic ulcer symptoms
Acute pericarditis	Costochondritis/musculoskeletal disorders
Aortic aneurysm	Pulmonary hypertension
Mitral valve prolapse	
Cardiac syndrome X	

Fig. 19 Differential diagnosis of chest pain.

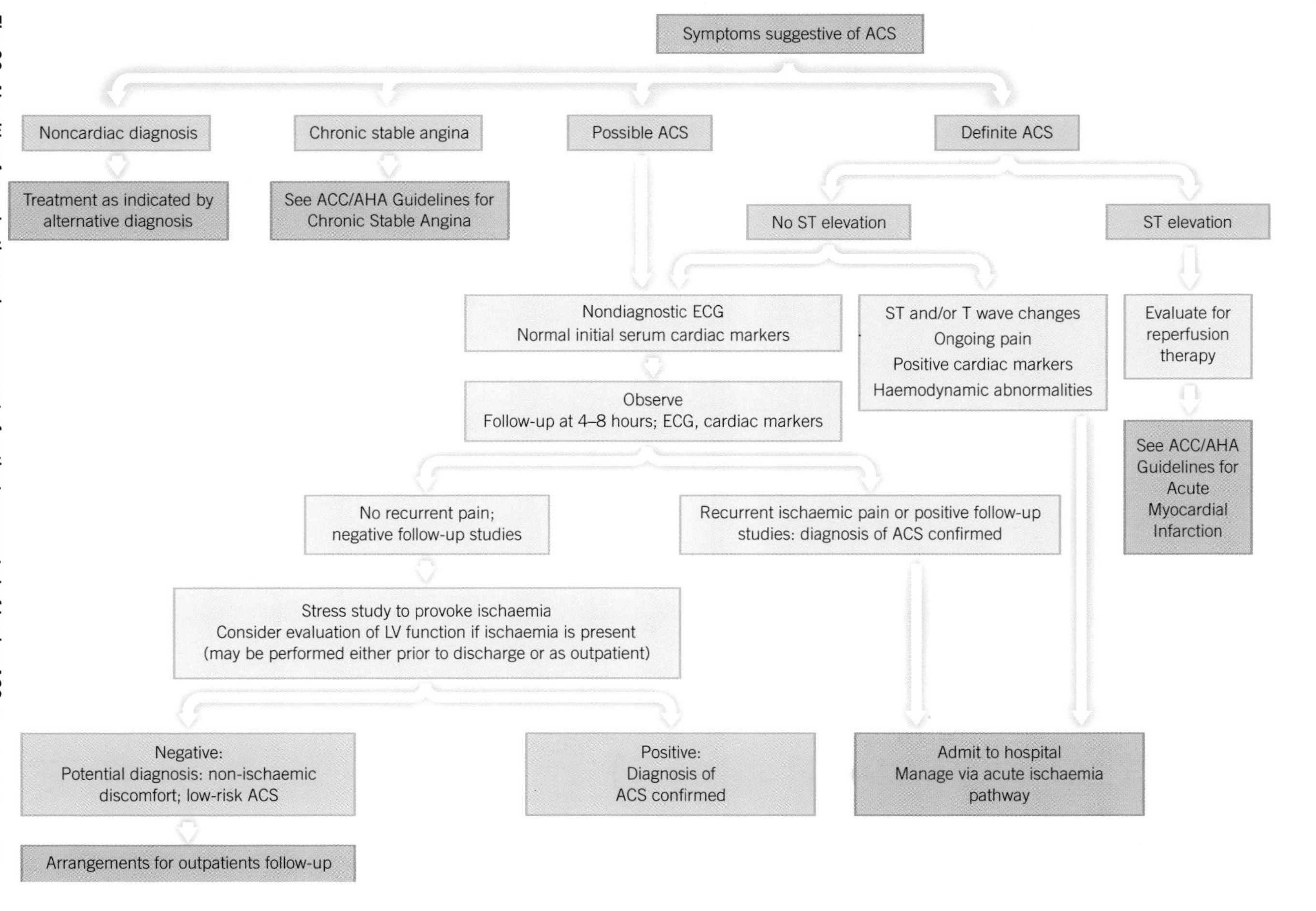

Fig. 20 Algorithm for evaluation and management of patients suspected of having ACS. Reproduced with permission from Committee on the Management of Patients with Unstable Angina. ACC/AHA guidelines for the management of patients with unstable angina and non-ST-segment elevation myocardial infarction. J Am Coll Cardiol 2000;36:970–1062. © Elsevier

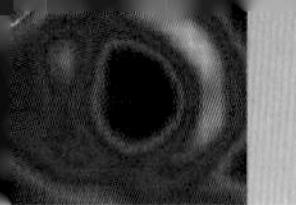

"Ischaemic ST changes and/or T wave inversion occurs commonly in patients with UA and usually resolves with relief of pain"

An algorithm for the evaluation and management of patients suspected of having ACS is provided in Figure 20.[28] Management of patients with definite STEMI will be addressed later.

Electrocardiography

A resting ECG should be obtained in all patients who present with chest pain. While the ECG is normal in about one third of chest pain patients, the presence of acute ischaemic changes on the admission ECG is associated with a higher risk of cardiac events. The pattern of ST and T wave abnormalities defines ACS patients as UA/NSTEMI versus STEMI (Figures 21a and 21b). This distinction affects both prognosis and therapeutic strategy. The ECG is seldom normal but may be equivocal in the early stages of an acute MI. Repeated recordings should be made and compared with earlier timed ECG strips. Severe ischaemia from UA/NSTEMI may be associated with transient ST elevation, whereas the ST elevation in STEMI persists for hours. In some cases of UA and NSTEMI the ST segments are normal, even during pain, with development of T wave inversion a few hours later. ECG findings further determine risk in ACS. In-hospital death has been reported as 8.7% with non-specific ECG changes and 11.5% with diagnostic results. Even a normal ECG carries a 5.7% 7-day mortality.[30]

New or reversible ST-segment deviation of 0.5 mm from baseline or left bundle branch block on the admission ECG is associated with an increase in incidence of death or MI at 1 year, i.e. 15.8 % versus

Fig. 21a NSTEMI in a 78-year-old man with chest pain. Troponin positive. Note: ST depression in V2 to V6 and to a lesser degree in I, II and aVF.

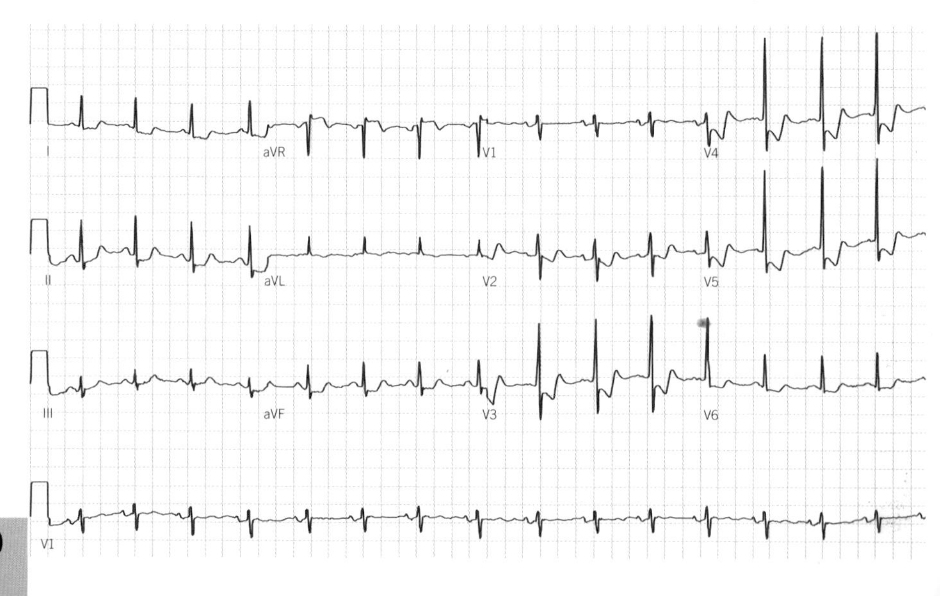

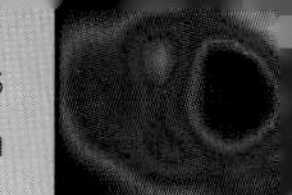

8.2% in patients without ECG changes.[31] Reversible ST-segment depression is associated with a 3- to 6-fold increase in death, MI, ischaemia at rest, or provocable ischaemia on exercise.[32] The ECG result and the CK level on admission can identify a difference in mortality (in the group with ST-segment elevation plus depression and elevated CK level).[33]

Ideally all suspected ACS patients should be admitted to the coronary care unit or monitored ward for 12 to 24 hours of ST-segment monitoring. The absence of ischaemic events during this period indicates a good prognosis. In contrast, prolonged or repeated ischaemic events indicate increased risk of future events.

Although not used routinely, continuous ambulatory ST-segment (Holter) monitoring can be a valuable tool for risk assessment. Patients with frequent transient episodes of ST-segment depression (the majority of which may occur silently) are at increased risk of adverse outcomes.[34]

"An elevated admission CK is associated with poor outcomes"

"The continuing presence of myocardial ischaemia on treadmill testing or Holter monitoring is associated with adverse outcomes"

Cardiac enzymes and biomarkers

Standard blood testing for the patient with suspected ACS in most hospitals includes TnI or TnT, total CK and CK-MB fraction. Increased serum levels of total CK and its MB isoenzyme are widely used for detection of MI, but these markers are neither cardiac specific for MI nor sensitive for identification of very small areas of myocardial necrosis. CK or CK-MB are not elevated until 3 to 4 hours post chest pain onset for MI (NSTEMI and STEMI) and are only poor

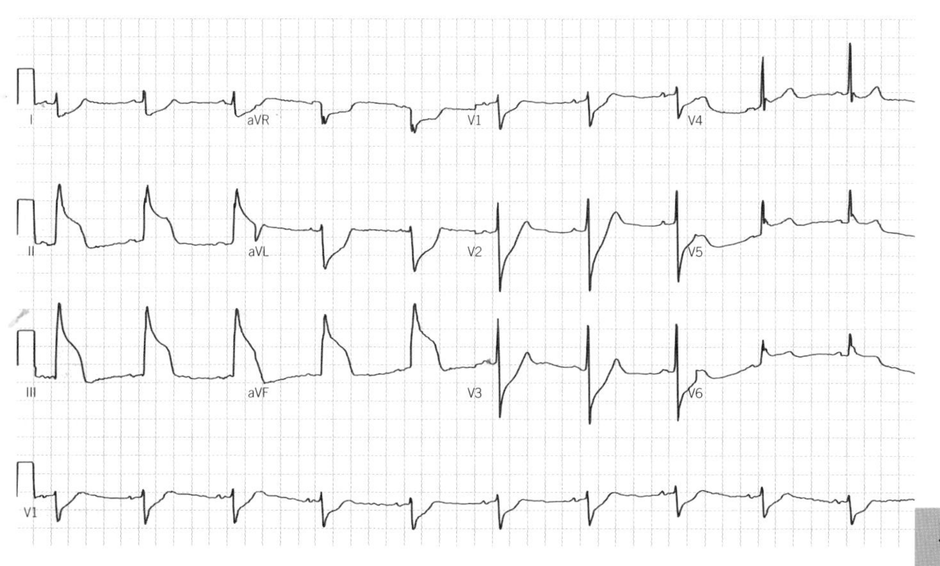

Fig. 21b Acute inferior MI in a 50-year-old man. Huge ST elevation in II, III and aVF and reciprocal changes in other leads.

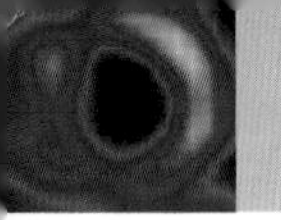

predictors of outcome. Elevated serum MB is an early marker of MI with detection as early as an hour after onset of myocardial injury. In some emergency departments MB testing is used to diagnose ACS although "positive" MB has poor specificity for myocardial damage, however normal MB is helpful to "rule out" MI. In contrast, cardiac isoforms of TnT and TnI are more specific and sensitive indicators of myocardial damage and can detect the micro-infarctions typified by NSTEMI. Both TnT and TnI can now be measured as a rapid assay and results should be available within 1 hour of blood draw allowing quick triage of patients into UA versus MI (either NSTEMI or STEMI) categories. TnT or TnI should be measured on admission and, if normal, repeated 6 to 12 hours later.

"In patients with suspected ACS, troponins should be measured on admission and, if normal, repeated 6–12 hours later"

There appears little to choose between cTnT and cTnI[35] however, as there are several commercial assays available for cTnI and not all give the same result or show equal sensitivity, it is best that both general practitioners and hospital physicians become aware of the assays used by their local laboratory, the sensitivity and reproducibility of the tests and the cut-off for diagnosis of MI.

Similar to CK, troponins are not very early markers of MI with serum increases starting around 4 hours post onset of pain. Studies of TnT versus TnI indicate that the two markers are equally sensitive and specific, and have similar prognostic significance. Negative troponins indicate low risk and predict reduced benefit from low molecular weight heparin (LMWH), GP IIb/IIIa receptor blockers, and routine invasive strategy.

"Physicians should be aware of the types of troponin assay used locally and their defined ranges"

MB and/or CK-MB mass may be measured in patients with recent (<6 hours) symptoms as an earlier marker of MI and in patients with recurrent ischaemia after recent (<2 weeks) infarction to detect further evidence.

Risk stratification

In addition to specific diagnosis of ACS, clinical investigations have been developed to assess risk of adverse cardiac events. Using the validated risk score from the TIMI study group, patients with UA/NSTEMI can be categorized into high-, intermediate- or low-risk groups determining treatment strategy and prognosis. The score is derived from seven standard clinical characteristics (below) routinely obtained during the initial medical evaluation in ACS patients. Each is assigned a value of 1 when present and 0 when absent. TIMI risks include:

- age >65
- ≥3 traditional risk factors for CAD (male sex, hyperlipidaemia, hypertension, smoking, diabetes mellitus, family history of premature CAD)

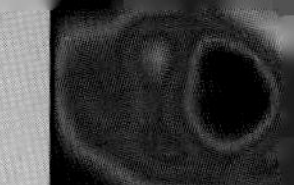

- prior coronary stenosis >50%
- ST segment elevation or depression at presentation
- ≥2 anginal events in the prior 24 hours
- aspirin use in the prior 7 days
- elevated serum cardiac biomarkers.

Feature	High risk (At least 1 of the following features must be present)	Intermediate risk (No high-risk feature but may have any of the following features)	Low risk (No high- or intermediate-risk feature but may have any of the following features)
History	Accelerating tempo of ischaemic symptoms in preceding 48 hours	Prior MI, peripheral or cerebrovascular disease, or CABG; prior aspirin use	
Character of pain	Prolonged (>20 min) rest pain	Prolonged (>20 min) rest angina, now resolved, with moderate or high likelihood of CAD Rest angina (<20 min or relieved with rest or sub-lingual glyceryl trinitrate)	New-onset or progressive CCS Class III or IV angina in the past 2 weeks with moderate or high likelihood of CAD
Clinical findings	Pulmonary oedema, most likely related to ischaemia New or worsening MR murmur S_3 or new/worsening rales Hypotension, bradycardia, tachycardia Age >75 years	Age >70 years	
ECG findings	Angina at rest with transient ST-segment changes >0.05 mV Bundle-branch block, new or presumed new Sustained ventricular tachycardia	T-wave inversions >0.2 mV Pathological Q-waves	Normal or unchanged ECG during an episode of chest discomfort
Cardiac markers	Elevated (e.g. TnT or TnI >0.1 ng/mL)	Slightly elevated (e.g. TnT >0.01 but <0.1 ng/mL)	Normal

CCS = Canadian Cardiovascular Society MR = mitral regurgitation

Fig. 22 Short-term risk of death or nonfatal MI in patients with UA. Reproduced with permission from ACC/AHA pocket guideline update. Management of patients with unstable angina and non-ST-segment elevation myocardial infarction. A report of the American College of Cardiology/American Heart Association Task Force on Practice Guidelines.

"Risk assessment can be performed based on clinical, ECG and biochemical data and a further treatment strategy can be selected"

TIMI risk score can be used to define high risk (≥5 points), intermediate risk (3–4 points), and low risk (0–2 points).[36] NSTEMI ACS patients with high or intermediate risk warrant aggressive pharmacologic and interventional treatment (Figure 22) whereas the low-risk cohort can be stabilized with a simple regimen. Along with TIMI, risk scores from the PURSUIT study and GRACE registry have been assessed.[37] PURSUIT uses a grading of 0 to 18, and GRACE 0 to 258 including heart rate, creatinine and Killip class. All appear to show good discriminatory accuracy in predicting major adverse cardiac events at both 30 days and 1 year. GRACE was best for predicting risk of death/MI at 1 year after admission. Figure 23 shows the criteria for stratification of ACS patients into high-risk and low-risk categories defined by the ESC,[35] which broadly concur with US classifications.

"The TIMI risk score is a validated way to assess risk of cardiac events"

Most data on risk stratification following acute MI are derived from studies done in the prethrombolytic era. Less information is available regarding risk stratification of patients treated with thrombolysis or primary angioplasty.[38]

Early risk stratification based on prethrombolytic criteria suggested that major determinants of mortality after acute MI include:

Fig. 23 Criteria for stratification of ACS patients. Based upon ESC Guidelines[35]

Risk stratification
From history, physical examination, ECG monitoring, blood samples

High-risk patients
Patients with recurrent ischaemia
Recurrent chest pain
Dynamic ST-segment changes (ST-segment depression or transient ST-segment elevation)
Early post infarction unstable angina
Elevated troponin levels
Diabetes
Haemodynamic instability
Major arrhythmias (VF, VT)

Low-risk patients
No recurrence of chest pain within observational period
No elevation of troponins or other markers of thrombosis
No ST-segment depression
Negative or flat T-waves, normal ECG

Second negative troponin measurement (6–12 hours)

- amount of myocardial necrosis
- residual myocardial ischaemia
- electrical instability
- three vessel CAD.

Approaches to management of acute MI will be addressed later on in this book (see pages 72–101).

"CRP is the best characterized of the current inflammatory biomarkers and has emerged as a marker of potential cardiovascular risk"

Inflammatory and other prognostic markers

As discussed above, inflammation has been recognized as an important feature of the pathophysiology of ACS. Recent data show that plasma markers of inflammation are useful risk predictors of ACS outcomes. CRP is a strong independent marker of increased cardiovascular risk in ACS.[39] hsCRP is also an independent predictor of risk of MI, stroke, peripheral vascular disease and sudden cardiac death even in apparently healthy individuals (Figure 24).[40] It has incremental prognostic value in association with levels of TnT. Patients with UA who have serum CRP levels over 1.5 mg/dL have a significantly worse outcome.

hsCRP adds prognostic information to all levels of LDL-cholesterol. In acute myocardial ischaemia hsCRP predicts poor outcome when troponin levels are normal, which suggests an enhanced inflammatory response is a factor in determining subsequent plaque rupture. There is no evidence yet that lowering CRP will lower vascular risk but weight loss and smoking cessation both lower CRP levels.

"BNP is a non-inflammatory biomarker that may be associated with a greater severity and extent of myocardial ischaemic territory during an ACS"

B-type natriuretic peptide (BNP) and NT-proBNP are non-inflammatory biomarkers released from ventricular myocardium in response to increased wall stress. Both BNP and NT-proBNP are elevated in ACS and both are independent risk predictors of mortality.[25] Importantly, elevated BNP and NT-proBNP reflect the extent of ischaemic myocardium at risk even when troponins, measures of necrosis, are normal or minimally elevated. Findings from the TACTICS-TIMI-18 trial[41] suggest that in patients with UA/NSTEMI, elevated levels of BNP (>80 pg/mL) are associated with tighter culprit stenosis and left anterior descending (LAD) coronary artery involvement during the index event.

New point of service (bedside) rapid tests are being developed to quantitate novel biomarkers permitting their future use in the acute care setting. Technical advances and additional clinical data hold out promise for future use of a multimarker strategy for risk assessment of ACS.

High risk	Intermediate risk	Low risk
>3 mg/L	1–3 mg/L	<1 mg/L

Fig. 24 hsCRP levels and associated risk.

Exercise testing

Exercise electrocardiography is the least expensive non-invasive test for myocardial ischaemia. Clearly exercise testing must *not* be considered during any unstable phase of CAD. Studies have however confirmed the safety and prognostic value of symptom-limited pre-discharge exercise testing in low-risk stabilized ACS patients with a normal resting ECG who are not taking digoxin.

“Exercise or pharmacological stress testing should be an integral part of evaluation of stabilized low-risk ACS patients”

Exercise, or (where appropriate) pharmacological, stress testing should ideally form a routine part of outpatient management. In this setting low risk could include patients with new-onset or progressive angina provoked by walking one block or one flight of stairs and who typically can be treated as outpatients.

Recommendations from the American Heart Association (AHA)[42] are that testing should be performed in most cases within 72 hours of presentation in low- or intermediate-risk individuals who are free of active ischaemia or heart failure symptoms for a minimum of 8–12 hours, and in intermediate-risk patients after 2–3 days. Selected patients can be evaluated earlier as part of a carefully constructed chest pain management protocol in, for example, a chest pain centre, after patients have been screened for high-risk features. In general the exercise treadmill test (Figure 25) should be the standard mode of stress testing in patients with a normal resting ECG who are not taking digoxin. Patients without ongoing symptoms with a normal ECG and a negative exercise test have an excellent prognosis. In

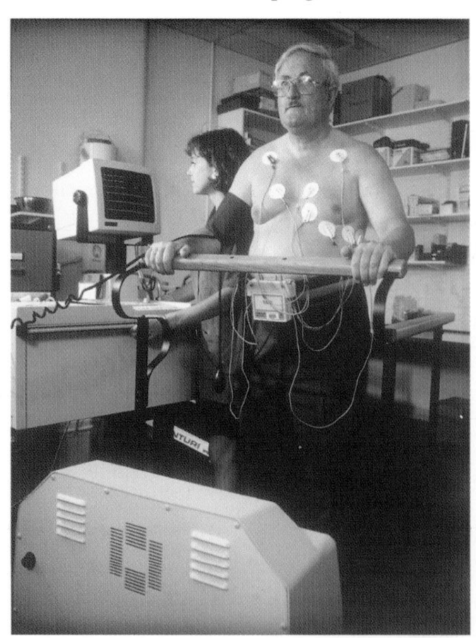

Fig. 25 The exercise treadmill test.

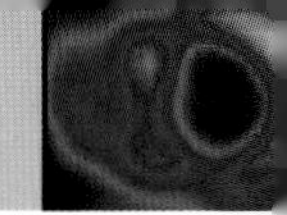

contrast, those patients who have a positive exercise test at an early stage, or who have widespread or prolonged ischaemia on the ECG, have a high risk of future events and should be considered for coronary angiography with a view to revascularization.

A recently reported substudy of DANAMI-2[43] describes the prognostic importance of a pre-discharge maximal exercise test following acute MI in the era of aggressive reperfusion treatment – thrombolysis and percutaneous coronary intervention (PCI). The prognostic significance of ST-segment depression seems to be strongest in the fibrinolysis treated patients.

A significant proportion of post-MI patients cannot perform an exercise test and in such cases an imaging technique such as perfusion scintigraphy or stress echocardiography increases sensitivity and specificity for prognosis.[35]

“In general the exercise treadmill should be the standard mode of testing”

Radionuclide imaging

Radionuclide myocardial perfusion imaging (MPI) is a robust technique for the assessment of patients with stable chronic chest pain with sensitivity and specificity for the detection of flow-limiting coronary stenosis in the region of 85–95% and 75–100%, respectively.[44] One of the greatest advantages of MPI is its ability to detect myocardial blood flow heterogeneity, one of the earliest events in the ischaemic cascade that occurs before functional and electrocardiographic abnormalities become manifested.

“Radionuclide MPI has a role to play in the early assessment and risk stratification of patients with ACS”

MPI in the assessment of acute chest pain

- *Thallium-201 imaging* Soon after its introduction in the mid 1970s as the first perfusion tracer for clinical use, the value of thallium-201 MPI for the diagnosis of ACS was investigated. It was observed that resting thallium-201 imaging was highly sensitive for the detection of acute myocardial hypoperfusion as well as very specific for the detection of areas of preserved myocardial blood flow.[45] Because thallium-201 redistributes soon after injection imaging should be completed within 30 minutes of injection to reflect myocardial distribution of thallium-201 at the time of administration. Late imaging will reflect the effect of redistribution with the potential for underestimation of the extent and severity of ischaemia. The need for a portable gamma camera to allow for immediate scanning as well as the potential for interfering with patient assessment and management have discouraged the use of thallium-201 in the acute setting.
- *Imaging with technetium-99m-labelled agents* The first studies evaluating the usefulness of acute technetium-99m MPI were

“Acute resting MPI is indicated in patients presenting to the emergency department with chest pain of suspected ischaemic origin but normal or nondiagnostic ECG”

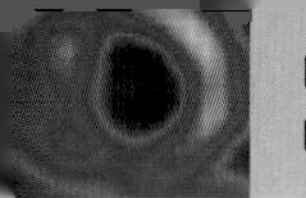

conducted soon after technetium-99m sestamibi became available in the early 1990s.[46] Technetium-99m sestamibi and technetium-99m tetrofosmin are taken up by the myocardium in proportion to blood flow, but unlike thallium-201, they exhibit long myocardial retention and slow washout with minimal redistribution over time, and thus imaging can be delayed for some time after injection. Technetium-99m-based tracers can be used to identify patients with acute myocardial ischaemia by injecting the tracer during ongoing symptoms and imaging up to several hours later without delaying management or compromising the diagnostic performance of the technique. If chest pain has abated at the time of evaluation the tracer can be administered up to 2 hours after resolution of symptoms bearing in mind that there is the potential for missing myocardial ischaemia if the tracer is given outside this time window.[47,48] A normal resting myocardial perfusion study has a high negative predictive value (99–100%)[46,49–52] for excluding acute MI and ischaemia, and thus rules out an ischaemic cause of chest pain in the acute setting (Figure 26). A normal scan is also

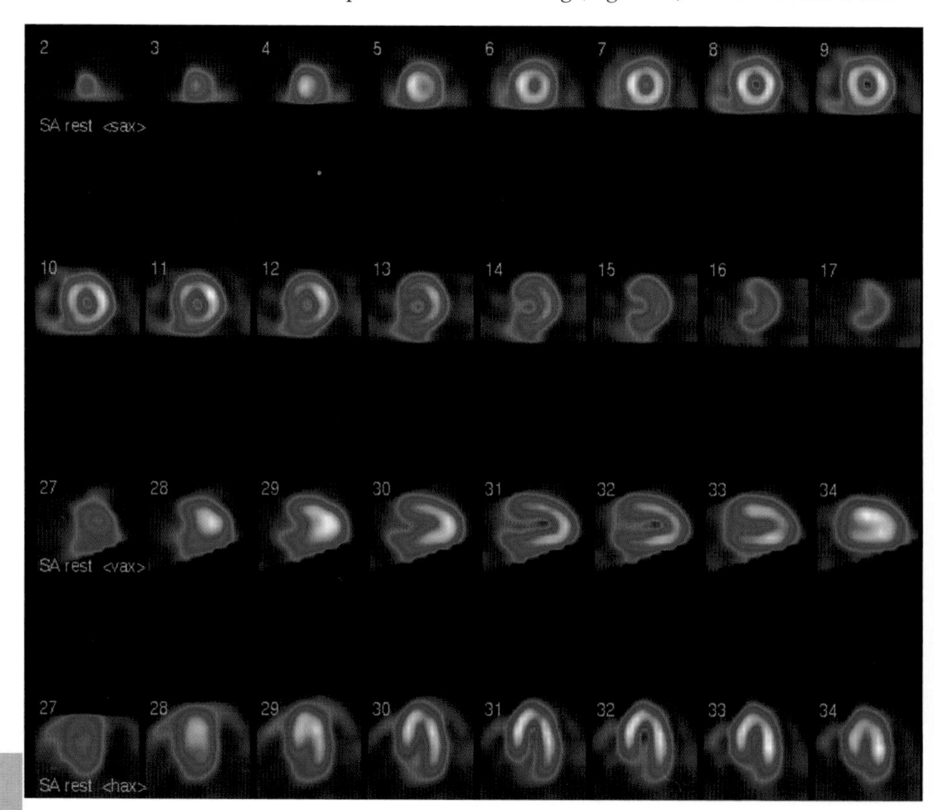

Fig. 26 Resting technetium-99m tetrofosmin myocardial perfusion SPECT study showing homogeneous distribution of tracer throughout the left ventricular myocardium. From top to bottom row: short-axis (sa), vertical long-axis (vla) and horizontal long-axis (hla) views.

associated with a relatively low likelihood of short- and medium-term cardiac events.[50] MPI therefore helps identify patients with a low probability of ACS who can be discharged home safely provided that further assessment with stress testing is conducted soon after discharge. In contrast an abnormal myocardial perfusion scan in a patient with acute chest pain and no history of previous MI is associated with a high probability of ACS and hospital admission is therefore mandatory.[49] A small proportion of patients will have equivocal, nearly normal or mildly abnormal acute resting MPI studies. These patients have been found to have an increased likelihood of acute coronary events compared with those with undoubtedly normal scans,[49] and thus a strategy of observation with serial measurement of serum cardiac biomarker levels and subsequent stress testing to rule out flow-limiting CAD is recommended for this group of patients.[47]

"Currently available perfusion tracers (e.g. thallium-201 and technetium-99m-labelled agents) distribute into viable myocardium in proportion to coronary blood flow and are not taken up by necrotic tissue, thus allowing the detection of acute ischaemia and infarction"

As for chronic stable chest pain, patients with an intermediate probability of ACS according to clinical and electrocardiographic criteria appear to benefit most from acute resting MPI.[28] Although a definite threshold for risk of ACS that warrants imaging has not been established, it is clear that patients with known CAD or multiple cardiovascular risk factors presenting with typical chest pain and ischaemic ECG changes have a high probability of ACS and thus would not benefit from acute imaging. Similarly, in patients with a very low likelihood of ACS MPI is unlikely to have an impact on outcome since the incidence of acute coronary events in this group is extremely low. In these patients early stress testing with or without imaging should be considered to rule out obstructive coronary disease.

Resting radionuclide imaging is of limited value in patients with history of CAD and documented previous MI as it is difficult to differentiate new acute MI or ongoing ischaemia from old infarction unless a previous MPI study is available for comparison. These patients also have a higher risk of cardiac events than their counterparts with no history of CAD, and thus resting perfusion imaging adds little diagnostic and prognostic information in this setting. By identifying patients who can be discharged safely from the emergency department or chest pain centres from those who require hospitalization acute resting MPI has the potential for reducing unnecessary hospital admissions and subsequent invasive diagnostic procedures, and may lead to substantial time saving with efforts allocated to the adequate management of patients with high probability or confirmed ACS. This was demonstrated by the largest published randomized trial that examined the feasibility and effectiveness of an emergency triage strategy that incorporated resting MPI in the initial assessment of

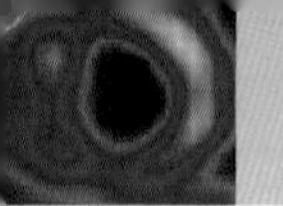

"A normal acute MPI study identifies low-risk patients eligible for safe discharge from the emergency room"

acute chest pain.[27] A significant reduction in the number of hospitalizations and diagnostic investigations was observed among patients without acute myocardial ischaemia in the imaging strategy arm. This approach did not affect the management of patients who were ultimately found to have ACS.[27] This acute imaging strategy may also prove to be cost-effective.[53] Controlled studies to assess this are on the way.

Detection of acute MI

After tracer injection, a positive MPI study can be demonstrated within 1 to 2 hours of acute myocardial injury. The presence of a resting perfusion abnormality has a high positive predictive value for acute MI in patients without prior infarction.[47] Conversely, a normal scan excludes acute myocardial injury but does not rule out the presence of flow-limiting coronary stenosis, and thus stress testing should be performed before or soon after hospital discharge for further assessment. Acute resting MPI provides earlier results than traditional serum biomarkers of myocardial injury with similar sensitivity for the detection of acute MI.[51,54] Because of the ability of the technique to provide information on both viability and regional myocardial blood flow at the time of injection, administration of tracer before and after thrombolysis or mechanical revascularization helps define the extent of jeopardized myocardium and myocardial salvage, which has prognostic value and has also been found to be highly useful in the evaluation of the effectiveness of new therapeutic interventions.

The limited spatial resolution of the technique implies that there is the potential for missing small subendocardial infarcts. Small subendocardial MIs are however associated with an uncomplicated clinical course and relatively good prognosis, and thus patients suspected to have experienced an acute MI should undergo further investigation with stress testing for the detection of residual ischaemia, assessment of prognosis and risk stratification.

Prognostic assessment after an ACS

- *MPI for risk stratification of patients with UA and NSTEMI* Stress MPI can be performed either after clinical stabilization or soon after discharge to guide further therapy and risk-stratify patients with UA or NSTEMI of uncomplicated course. MPI not only provides independent and incremental prognostic information but also identifies those patients most likely to benefit from coronary revascularization by defining the amount and extent of inducible ischaemia in the distribution of the culprit lesion as well as in the remote myocardium (Figure 27).[55,56]

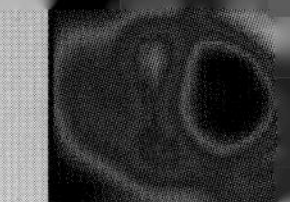

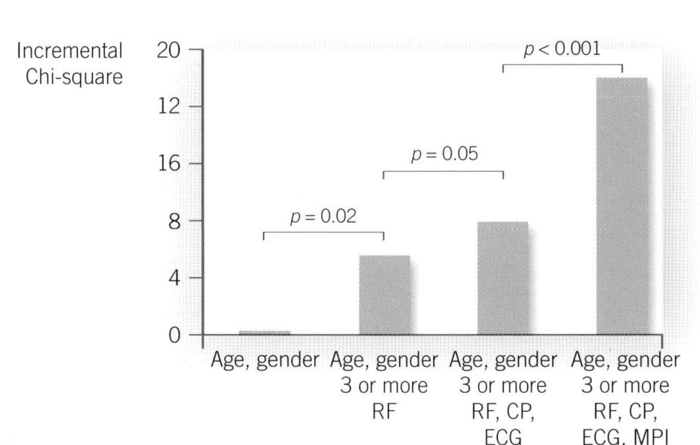

Fig. 27 Incremental prognostic information. Provided by demographic (age and gender), cardiovascular risk factors (RF), chest pain (CP), electrocardiographic (ECG) and myocardial perfusion imaging (MPI) variables shown by Chi-square in patients with suspected ACS but nondiagnostic ECG. Reproduced with permission from Heller GV, Stowers SA, Hendel RC, et al. Clinical value of acute rest technetium-99m tetrofosmin tomographic myocardial perfusion imaging in patients with acute chest pain and nondiagnostic electrocardiograms. J Am Coll Cardiol 1998;31:1011–1017. © Elsevier

- *MPI for risk stratification after acute STEMI* Following an uncomplicated acute MI evidence-based medicine and current clinical guidelines recommend stress testing for the assessment of the presence and magnitude of residual myocardial ischaemia that has both therapeutic and prognostic implications.[57,58] Stress testing is recommended in post acute MI patients with preserved left ventricular function who did not have coronary angiography as part of their initial management and in whom coronary revascularization would be considered.[57,58] In this setting MPI enables accurate assessment of the extent and severity of inducible ischaemia in the territory of the infarct-related artery, as well as in the remote myocardium, allowing the identification of patients with extensive coronary disease who are at high risk of cardiac events and thus are likely to benefit from mechanical revascularization. Patients with minimal or no evidence of inducible myocardial ischaemia can be treated medically.[59] Because its diagnostic performance is not affected by the type of stress test used MPI can be performed early (24–72 hours post-clinical stabilization) after an uncomplicated acute MI with the use of vasodilator agents (e.g. dipyridamole, adenosine),[60] which have demonstrated excellent safety profiles and high diagnostic accuracy for the detection of residual ischaemia.[61] The extent and

“Stress MPI provides valuable prognostic information that guides clinical-decision making regarding the need for revascularization and assists in risk stratification of post-ACS patients”

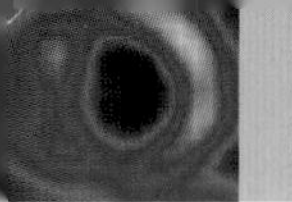

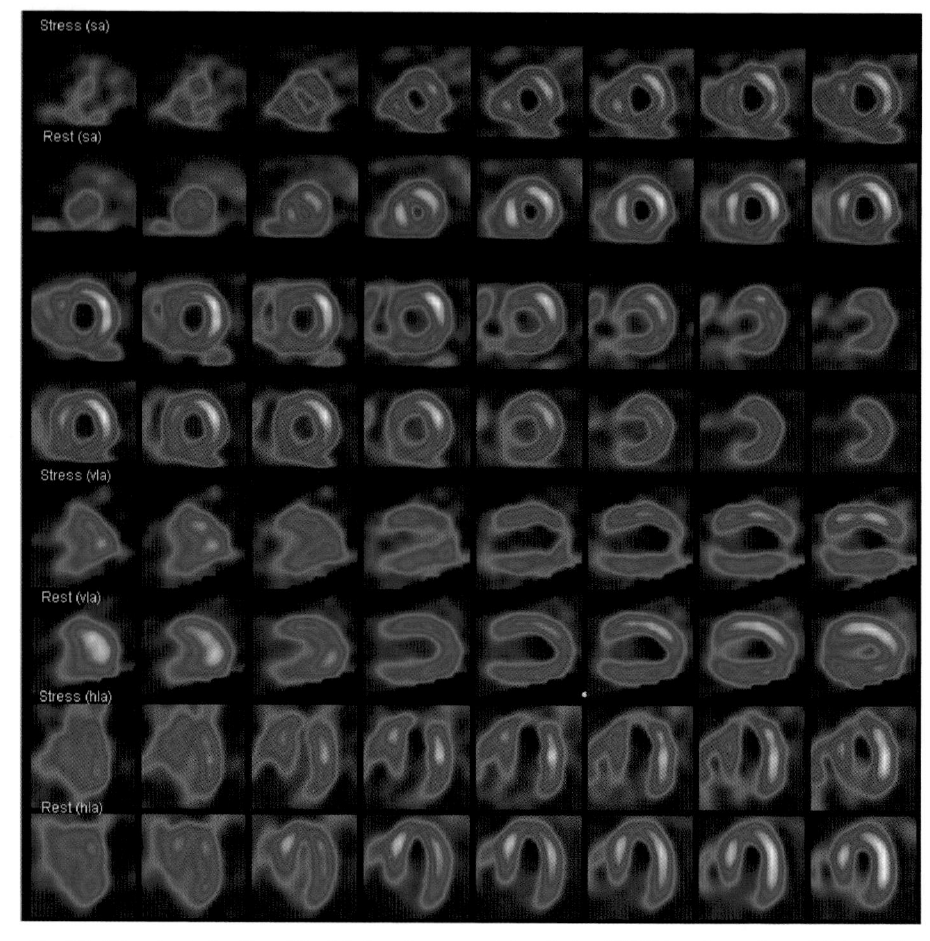

Fig. 28 Adenosine technetium-99m tetrofosmin myocardial perfusion SPECT imaging performed 4 days after an uncomplicated acute MI. The images show partial thickness inferior and apical MI with superimposed ischaemia. In addition there is evidence of inducible ischaemia in the anteroseptal region. From top to bottom row: short-axis (sa), vertical long-axis (vla) and horizontal long-axis (hla) views.

severity of stress-induced perfusion abnormalities as well as the magnitude of reversibility on pre-discharge imaging provide incremental prognostic information for early risk stratification of post acute MI patients (Figure 28).[52,61] According to previous studies, post acute MI patients with extensive and severe inducible perfusion abnormalities on stress MPI have an annual rate of cardiac death or nonfatal MI in the region of 12% compared with an event rate of 2% per year in those with small perfusion defects.[55,62]

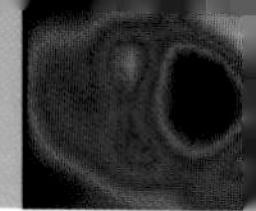

Simultaneous assessment of perfusion and left ventricular function by resting MPI

The prognostic value of left ventricular function in patients with CAD is well documented. In the acute setting left ventricular dysfunction is associated with a poor outcome. Simultaneous assessment of function and perfusion is possible with the use of ECG-gated acquisition after administration of high-energy tracers such as technetium-99m sestamibi and tetrofosmin. ECG gating not only provides incremental prognostic information and allows further risk stratification but also increases the specificity of the technique by means of the detection of defects resulting from attenuation artefact.[63,64]

“The extent and severity of perfusion abnormalities on MPI along with other non-perfusion variables such as transient left ventricular dilatation, increased lung tracer uptake and ventricular dysfunction on ECG-gating are important prognostic markers of risk of future cardiac events after an uncomplicated ACS”

Conclusion

MPI is a sensitive technique for the detection of acute abnormalities of myocardial blood flow that result from an imbalance between myocardial oxygen demand and supply. Even more important is its ability to accurately identify patients without acute ischaemia. A triage approach that includes resting perfusion imaging has been demonstrated to enhance clinical decision-making and patient management. Moreover MPI provides valuable diagnostic information that is available soon after initial assessment and enables the evaluation of patients with ongoing chest pain as well as resolved symptoms, overcoming the major limitations of serial cardiac enzyme analysis and echocardiography.[51,65,66] Randomized trials examining the impact of an imaging-based strategy for risk stratification of post acute MI patients as well as the cost-effectiveness of acute imaging are on the way.[67] Other nuclear techniques, including metabolic imaging with radio-labelled fluorodeoxyglucose (FDG) and fatty acid analogues (e.g. 15-(p-[iodine-123]iodophenyl)-3-(R,S) methylpentadecanoic acid or BMIPP), are currently under investigation as potential diagnostic tools for the early assessment of patients with suspected acute myocardial ischaemia.[68]

Echocardiography

Echocardiography is not used routinely in all hospitals to confirm diagnosis of ACS, although it may be particularly useful in patients with a non-diagnostic ECG and also to risk stratify patients. Both resting and stress echocardiography (echo) play an increasingly important role in the general assessment of CAD as ischaemia results in immediate changes that can be detected by echo.[69] These include:

- abnormalities of wall motion – hypokinetic, akinetic, dyskinetic (also known as asynergy)

Acute heart failure	Severe left ventricular impairment
Acute mitral regurgitation	Due to papillary muscle dysfunction or rupture
Acute ventricular septal defect	More common in inferior and right ventricular infarction
Mural thrombus	Usually located near infarcted segment or aneurysm
Left ventricular aneurysm	More common in anterior than inferior MI
Pseudoaneurysm	Rare, following rupture of left ventricular free wall
Pericardial effusion	Detected by M-mode or 2-D echo
Myocardial function post-MI	Gives an indication of prognosis

Fig. 29 Echo-assessed complications of acute MI.

- abnormalities of wall thickening – reduced or absent systolic thickening or systolic thinning
- abnormalities of overall left ventricular function – e.g. ejection fraction.

Left ventricular dysfunction, measured as reduced ejection fraction (<40%) or as a wall motion score index, is one of the major determinants of long-term risk.[9] All the above can be detected using 2-D echo but M-mode is also extremely good as the high sampling rate makes it very sensitive to wall motion and thickening abnormalities. It is essential that the ultrasound beam is at 90 degrees to the wall. There are limited regions of the left ventricular myocardium that can be examined by M-mode – most usefully the posterior wall and intraventricular septum.

“Echocardiography can identify severe hypokinesis or akinesis of an infarcted area, which may be helpful in patients with a non-diagnostic ECG”

Echo can provide rapid and non-invasive confirmation of the acute complications of MI, as shown in Figure 29. Scarred myocardium is seen as a thin segment that does not thicken during systole and has abnormal motion.

The changes in left ventricular function with MI are similar to those described for ischaemia but rapidly become irreversible. Detection of right ventricular involvement is important in determining treatment and prognosis. Measurement of ejection fraction or wall motion score index also allows for assessment and improvement in left ventricular function following successful reperfusion therapy (thrombolysis or primary angioplasty). It also helps identify high-risk patients who may benefit from early use of ACE inhibitors.

“Stress echo in patients who have stabilized, provides information on cardiac function and on the location and extent of jeopardized myocardium”

Stress echo can involve exercise or stress induced by pharmacologic agents, such as dipyridamole or dobutamine, to provoke ischaemia, which can be used to provide additional prognostic information in patients whose unstable symptoms have settled. A test is considered positive if wall motion abnormalities develop with stress in previously normal vascular territories or worsen in a segment that was abnormal

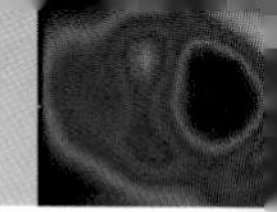

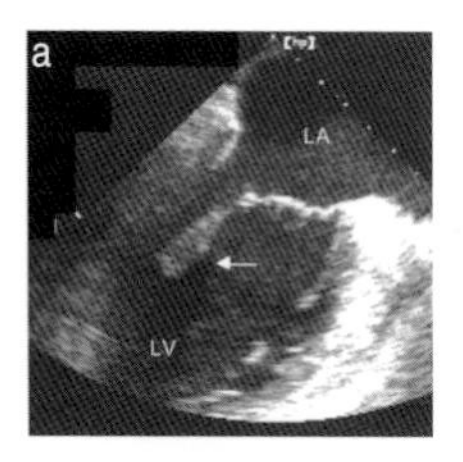

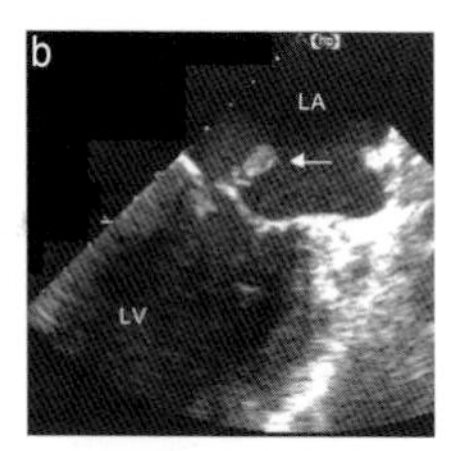

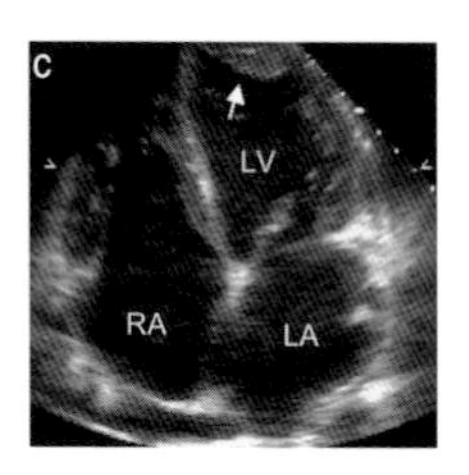

Originally published in: Kaddoura S. Echo Made Easy. Edinburgh: Churchill Livingstone, 2002.

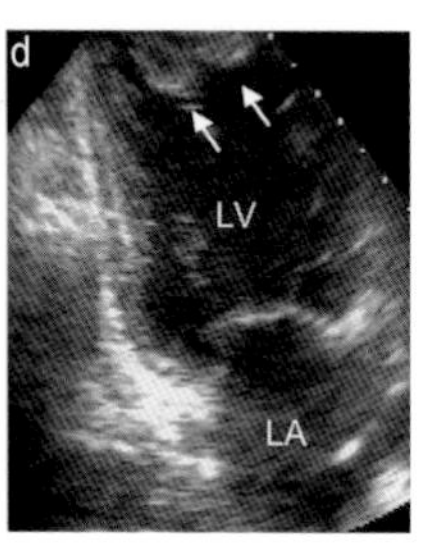

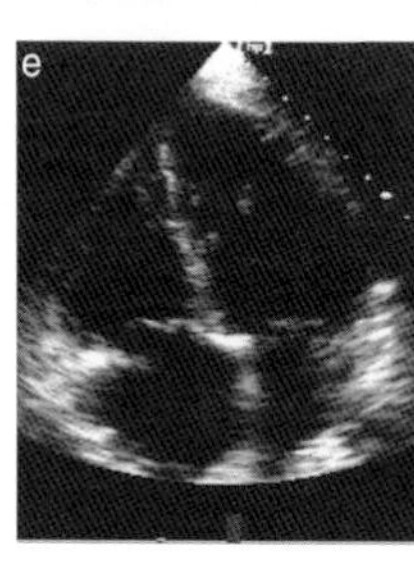

Fig. 30 Echocardiographs. a,b: Papillary muscle rupture following acute MI. The muscle (arrows) and the posterior mitral valve leaflet can be seen to prolapse into the left atrium. c,d: Thrombus in the apex of the LV (arrows) following MI: (c) apical 4-chamber view and (d) apical 2-chamber view showing two distinct masses. e: Dilated right ventricle (arrow) following acute RV infarction: apical 4-chamber view.

at baseline. As is true of radionuclide perfusion imaging, stress echo provides information on the location and extent of jeopardized myocardium. In addition this test provides insight into left ventricular and cardiac-valve function.

A newer technique, myocardial contrast echocardiography, allows accurate assessment of regional myocardial perfusion. It is performed by injection of microbubbles into the coronary circulation to differentiate perfused and non-perfused tissue, which may be useful in assessment of patients following reperfusion treatment.

“Coronary angiography remains the “gold standard” in defining coronary anatomy”

Coronary angiography

While coronary angiography is regarded as the “gold standard” to define coronary anatomy it does not provide functional information and it carries a small but definite mortality, i.e. 1 in 1400.[70] Coronary angiographic studies in UA have shown that multivessel disease is common. Analysis of lesion morphology shows a high prevalence of complex lesions with features of acute angulation with irregularity or intraluminal thrombus. Following maximal antianginal medication the continued development of transient ischaemia is strongly associated with these features and with poorer outcomes.[71] In UA patients who stabilize medically, subsequent short-term stenosis progression and coronary events are common.[72] This suggests that the presence of complete stenoses, even in patients who settle with medical treatment, calls for more urgent revascularization with angioplasty or bypass graft surgery. Diabetic patients with UA studied using coronary angioscopy have been shown to have a higher incidence of plaque ulceration and intracoronary thrombus than non-diabetic patients. This increase in

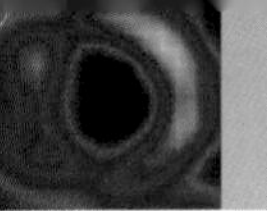

complex lesion morphology is likely to account for the disproportionately higher risk for development of ACS in these patients.[73]

"While high-risk patients should undergo urgent cardiac catheterization, many low-risk patients may also benefit from this investigation"

Coronary angiography should be performed in patients where the diagnosis cannot be reliably made using non-invasive testing. Patients with high-risk clinical markers, who tend to be older, have multiple risk factors and have previous MI, should undergo early coronary angiography. (Cardiac catheterization and intervention in STEMI will be discussed later, see pages 80–101.) Likewise, patients at high risk by imaging criteria, i.e. reduced ejection fraction, or those with extensive or profound inducible ischaemia should also undergo coronary angiography.

Similarly, high-risk UA patients who are refractory to medical therapy should be referred urgently for angiography with a view to intervention. A relatively small group require angiography within the first hour of hospital admission; these include those patients with severe ongoing ischaemia, major arrhythmias and haemodynamic instability. In most cases however, angiography is performed within 24 hours or at least during the hospitalization period.[35] Recommendations for the choice of revascularization in UA are similar to those for elective revascularization procedures.

Coronary angiography is also warranted in some patients considered to be at low risk for rapid progression to MI or death. These include patients with chronic stable symptoms who experience "break through" angina or who fail medical therapy in addition to those who develop significant ischaemia on exercise testing at low workloads. Younger patients (below age 50) may also benefit from angiography as they may have advanced or significant cardiac anomalies and/or multivessel disease.

While there has historically been under-provision of coronary angiography in the UK and other countries, there is evidence that services are increasing and rates are currently rising.

Conclusions

As we have shown, there are numerous tests and markers to identify myocardial ischaemia and abnormal biochemistry in patients with a suspected ACS. No single test or strategy is definitive. However the clinical history and physical examination coupled with the 12-lead ECG and troponin/CK-MB measurement provides sufficient information to establish a diagnosis in most patients. This information may be supplemented with imaging and coronary angiography to guide the physician in the appropriate management and risk stratification of the patient thereafter.

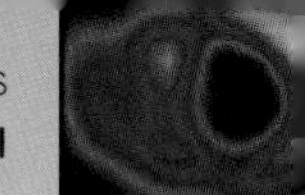

Management of UA/NSTEMI

General treatment guidelines

The use of combination evidence-based medical treatments including antiplatelet agents, beta-blockers, statins and ACE inhibitors has been shown to be independently and strongly associated with lower 6-month mortality in patients with ACS.[74] Such findings suggest that following accepted protocols, in keeping with initiatives such as "Get with the Guidelines" from the AHA, helps ensure continuous quality improvement of heart attack treatment and prevention. It also focuses on care team protocols to ensure that patients are treated and discharged appropriately.

"Application of current evidence-based guidelines significantly improves outcomes in patients with ACS"

Workers have also assessed the treatment effect of combined therapy in ACS patients stratified according to their risk of future cardiovascular events according to their TIMI risk score (see pages 32–35).[75] Combination evidence-based medical treatment was associated with lower 6-month mortality in patients with ACS, with a gradient of benefit across the different TIMI risk groups.

"Application of conventional guidelines is suboptimal, perhaps because of their length and complexity"

Despite this, implementation of formal guidelines remains suboptimal. There may be several reasons for this related to lack of awareness, familiarity or agreement with the guideline recommendations. Their length and complexity may also play a role. In order to address this issue Gluckman and colleagues have devised a simplified "ABCDE" comprehensive approach.[76] The elements include:

- A for antiplatelet therapy, anticoagulation, ACE inhibition or angiotensin receptor blockade (see pages 52–62, 62–67, 117–119)
- B for beta-blockade and blood pressure control (see pages 50–51, 117)
- C for cigarette smoking cessation and cholesterol treatment (see pages 110–117)
- D for diet and diabetes management (see pages 110–117, 119–120)
- E for exercise (see page 121).

"A simplified ABCDE approach is now available to more effectively create management protocols and ensure implementation of risk-reducing treatment strategies"

This simple ABCDE evidence-based approach (modified from guidelines from the ACC/AHA) allows physicians and hospitals to create disease management protocols and to define roles and responsibilities for different medical personnel in order to ensure implementation of short- and long-term strategies to reduce risk. The ABCDE approach is summarized in Figure 31. The evidence for the various recommendations can be found within the sections that follow.

Anti-ischaemic therapies

Nitrates

Treatment with sublingual or intravenous (iv) nitrates is routine in patients with ACS. They are used despite the lack of any convincing

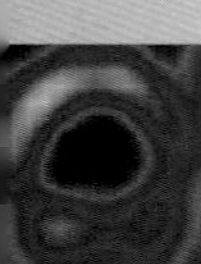

	Intervention	Agent(s)/treatment modalities	Comments
A	Antiplatelet therapy	Aspirin	All patients indefinitely Initially with 162–325 mg followed by 75–160 mg daily thereafter (outside US, use dosages as recommended by local protocols)
		ADP receptor antagonist (clopidogrel)	All patients, unless anticipated need for urgent CABG surgery or within 5 days of electively scheduled CABG surgery Duration of up to 1 year
		GP IIb/IIIa inhibitor (abciximab, eptifibatide, tirofiban)	All patients with continuing ischaemia, an elevated troponin level, a TIMI risk score >4, or anticipated PCI Avoid abciximab if PCI is not planned
	Anticoagulation	Unfractionated heparin	Alternative to LMWH for patients managed with an early invasive strategy
		LMWH (specifically enoxaparin)	Preferred anticoagulant if managed conservatively Alternative to unfractionated heparin for patients managed with an early invasive strategy Avoid if creatinine clearance is <60 mL/min (unless anti-Xa levels are to be followed) or CABG surgery within 24 hours
	ACE inhibition	No clear preferred agent	All patients with left ventricular systolic dysfunction (ejection fraction <40%), heart failure, hypertension, or other high-risk features
	Angiotensin receptor blockade	No clear preferred agent	All patients intolerant of ACE inhibitors Avoid combination therapy with ACE inhibitors acutely, but consider in patients with chronic left ventricular systolic dysfunction (ejection fraction <40%) and heart failure
B	Beta-blockade	No clear preferred agent	All patients
	Blood pressure control	ACE inhibitors and beta-blockers first line	Goal at least <130/85 mmHg (<130/80 mmHg if diabetes or chronic kidney disease present) Optimal may be as low as 125/75 mmHg
C	Cholesterol treatment	Potent high-dose statin	All patients Goal LDL < 70 mg/dL
		Ezetimibe or bile acid sequestrant (resin)	All patients unable to achieve an LDL level <70 mg/dL while taking a potent high-dose statin
		Fibrates or nicotinic acid (niacin)	Consider in patients with HDL <40 mg/dL or triglycerides >150 mg/dL while taking a potent high-dose statin
	Cigarette smoking cessation	Long-term behavioural support Bupropion plus nicotine replacement	All patients using tobacco
D	Diabetes management	Glycaemic control – HbA_{1c} <7% (minimum)	All patients with diabetes
	Diet	Weight reduction to achieve optimal body mass index Dietary modification	All patients
E	Exercise	Aerobic and weight-bearing exercise 4–5 times per week for >30 minutes	All patients preferably within a cardiac rehabilitation programme

Fig. 31 ABCDEs of cardiovascular disease management in UA/NSTEMI. Reproduced with permission from Gluckman TJ, Sachdev M, Schulman SP, Blumenthal RS. A simplified approach to the management of non-ST-segment elevation acute coronary syndromes. JAMA 2005;293:349–357. © American Medical Association. Adapted from ACC/AHA guidelines.

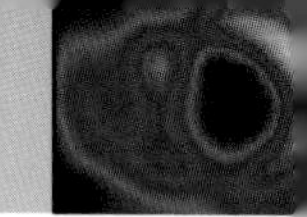

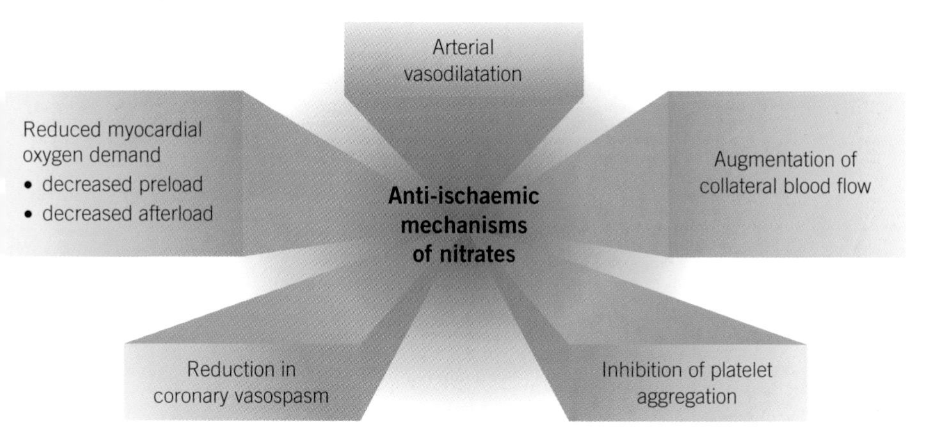

Fig. 32 Anti-ischaemic mechanisms of nitrates.

data that they reduce mortality or reinfarction.[31] Their main role is to provide relief of pain. Their anti-ischaemic effects are shown in Figure 32.

Intravenous glyceryl trinitrate (nitroglycerin) is routinely administered to hospitalized ACS patients. This is titrated up until symptoms are relieved or side effects occur, most notably headache or hypotension. There are no data to indicate the optimal intensity or duration of nitrate use.[35] Tolerance may develop after 24 hours of use but the mechanism of this is poorly understood. The potassium channel activator, nicorandil, is an alternative nitrate-like drug, although it is not available in all countries.

“Nitrates are routinely used for relief of pain in ACS”

Nicorandil

Nicorandil is available in some countries for the treatment of angina and to reduce the frequency of events in individuals with chronic stable angina. It is a hybrid compound comprising a potassium channel opener with a nitrate moiety.[77] Nicorandil has dual mechanisms of action on both preload and afterload producing a dose-related improvement in haemodynamics. Nicorandil may mimic ischaemic preconditioning, which is a powerful protection against myocardial necrosis. Unlike classical nitrates there appears to be an absence of haemodynamic tolerance to nicorandil. Nicorandil appears to have comparable efficacy and tolerability to other standard antianginals.

“There is no convincing evidence that nitrates reduce rates of death or reinfarction”

There is limited experience with nicorandil in acute MI and it is not used routinely in this setting. An initial small study conducted in 245 patients with UA[78] demonstrated that the addition of nicorandil to standard therapy with nitrates, beta-blockers, diltiazem, aspirin and heparin, reduced ischaemic episodes and tachyarrhythmias compared with placebo. This led to further larger investigations in a stable angina

“Nicorandil is a nitrate-like drug, available in some countries”

"Nicorandil is not used routinely, but may have a role to further reduce ischaemia in ACS"

population. The IONA[79] study showed that nicorandil 20 mg twice daily, in addition to standard antianginal therapy, improved outcomes in terms of reducing events related to acute coronary disease and the associated requirement for admission to hospital. The drug may therefore have a useful role in the treatment of angina that is unresponsive to initial medical treatment.

Beta-blockers

Patients with ACS without ST-segment elevation, who do not have contraindications, should be treated with beta-blockers as soon as possible to prevent acute MI/reinfarction.[35,80] Similarly, oral beta-blockers are recommended for long-term use, indefinitely, in all patients who recover from an acute MI. Beta-blockers afford cardio-protection through a number of mechanisms including preventing cardiac rupture, reinfarction, sudden cardiac death and ventricular arrhythmias. The prevention of the cardiotoxic effects of catecholamines plays a central role, reducing sympathetic drive and myocardial ischaemia. Beta-blockers decrease myocardial oxygen demand by reducing heart rate, cardiac contractility, and systolic blood pressure. Beta-blockers may also improve cardiac function because they prolong diastolic filling and coronary diastolic perfusion time. Their antiarrhythmic effects result from direct cardiac electrophysiological activity with reduced heart rate, decreased spontaneous firing of ectopic pacemakers, slowed conduction and increased refractory period of the atrioventricular (AV) node.

"Beta-blockers should be used in all ACS patients (in absence of contraindications) as soon as possible"

Meta-analysis of randomized controlled trials after MI shows that beta-blockers reduce the odds of death in long-term trials by 23% and in short-term trials by 4%.[81] A study in nearly 70,000 patients prescribed beta-blockers (atenolol, metoprolol, propranolol) following acute MI[82] showed that these agents were associated with a 40% improvement in survival at 2 years, and suggested that the specific beta-blocker chosen will have little influence on mortality. Improvements were seen compared with placebo whether or not the drugs were cardioselective or non-selective (Figure 33). Although the evidence of benefit for beta-blockers in UA is limited, because of the similar pathophysiology of UA and acute MI, these agents are uniformly recommended as first-line treatment for all ACS.

"While there are few studies in UA there are persuasive data from studies of beta-blockers in acute MI"

Most evidence is available for propranolol, timolol and metoprolol, and it cannot be assumed that prognostic benefit will be achieved with other agents. Although atenolol is widely used it has been inadequately evaluated.

There are no large long-term studies assessing the effects of beta-blockers on mortality in patients with stable angina pectoris.[83]

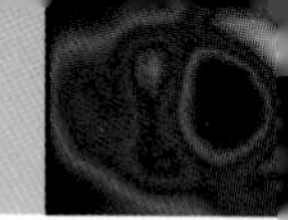

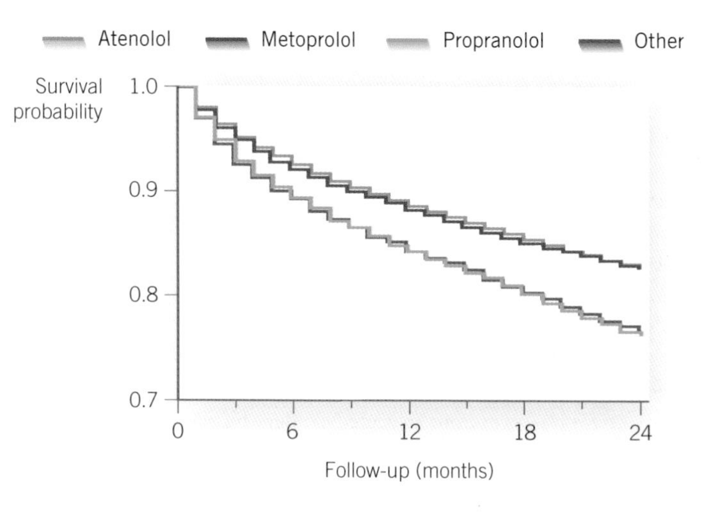

Fig. 33 Unadjusted mortality of patients receiving different beta-blockers after MI.

Reproduced with permission from Gottlieb SS, McCarter RJ. Comparative effects of three beta blockers (atenolol, metoprolol, and propranolol) on survival after acute myocardial infarction. Am J Cardiol 2001;87:823–826. © Elsevier

Similarly most of the large beta-blocker trials were performed in the prethrombolysis era, and there is also little information on the role of beta-blockers used with aspirin and/or statins. Beta-blockers can cause a variety of adverse effects, notably fatigue and extreme bradycardia, as well as interfering with respiratory function, which can cause some patients not to tolerate them. Some 20% of patients do not respond to any beta-blocker[84] necessitating the switch to a heart rate lowering calcium antagonist, e.g. diltiazem.

> *"There are no large long-term studies assessing the effects of beta-blockers on mortality in patients with stable angina pectoris"*

Calcium antagonists

The antianginal effects of calcium antagonists appear to be mediated through a reduction of myocardial oxygen demand secondary to decreased afterload and myocardial contractility.[85] There are three main classes:

- dihydropyridines, e.g. nifedipine, amlodipine
- non-dihydropyridines – verapamil and diltiazem classes.

All of these agents are effective antianginals but because dihydropyridines may cause reflex tachycardia they are normally prescribed with a beta-blocker in stable angina patients. Diltiazem may cause bradycardia while verapamil can also cause significant depression of myocardial contractility necessitating caution when used with beta-blockade. These latter two agents should not be used in patients with pulmonary congestion/heart failure or AV dysfunction.

There is evidence that calcium antagonists may retard the atherosclerotic process,[86] but more complete clinical data are required to establish whether calcium antagonists have any role other than symptom control in patients with angina. A meta-analysis of trials of patients with acute MI or UA who were treated with calcium antagonists found that these agents do not reduce the risk of initial or recurrent infarction or death.[87] In the HINT trial[88] in patients who were not previously receiving beta-blockers, conventional nifedipine was associated with a 16% higher risk of MI/recurrent angina versus placebo; whereas the combination of nifedipine/metoprolol was associated with a 20% lower incidence of these events (neither reached statistical significance). This may be explained by the reflex tachycardia produced by nifedipine as monotherapy. Nifedipine and other dihydropyridines should not therefore be used in ACS without beta-blockade, and then only as third-line treatment in refractory ischaemia, using oral and long-acting preparations, with beta-blockers and nitrates. Heart rate lowering calcium antagonists offer an alternative when patients cannot tolerate a beta-blocker although caution is urged when combining the two.[89]

“There is no role for calcium antagonists in the acute phase of STEMI”

There has been considerable controversy about the overall safety of calcium antagonists but the Blood Pressure Lowering Treatment Trialists Collaboration overview[90] and ACTION[91] have established the safety of this drug class in chronic stable angina. The INTERCEPT study showed the safety, and to some degree the benefit, of diltiazem in patients with acute MI but without heart failure who had received thrombolysis.[92] Diltiazem was associated with a relative decrease in the combined event rate for non-fatal MI and refractory ischaemia. There is however no case for using calcium antagonists prophylactically in the acute phase of MI.[57]

Oral antiplatelet therapies

The important biological role of platelets in atherothrombosis has resulted in a number of trials of oral antiplatelet therapy for the management of ACS. The first antiplatelet agent to be used widely was aspirin, which reduces death or recurrent MI by 50% in patients with UA or NSTEMI and produces a 23% reduction in cardiovascular death among patients with STEMI. A better understanding of platelet biology has identified ADP as a key player in platelet activation and subsequent aggregation (Figure 34). Clopidogrel belongs to a new class of drugs called thienopyridines, which irreversibly block the P_2Y_{12} component of the ADP receptor for the duration of the life of the platelet (on average 5 days).

Aspirin

Acute treatment with aspirin is recommended in all patients with suspected ACS in the absence of contraindications.[35] An estimated 20–25 million Americans take aspirin daily for the prevention of life-

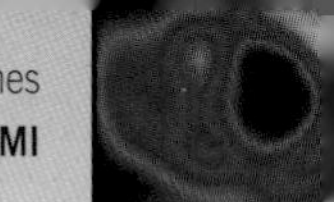

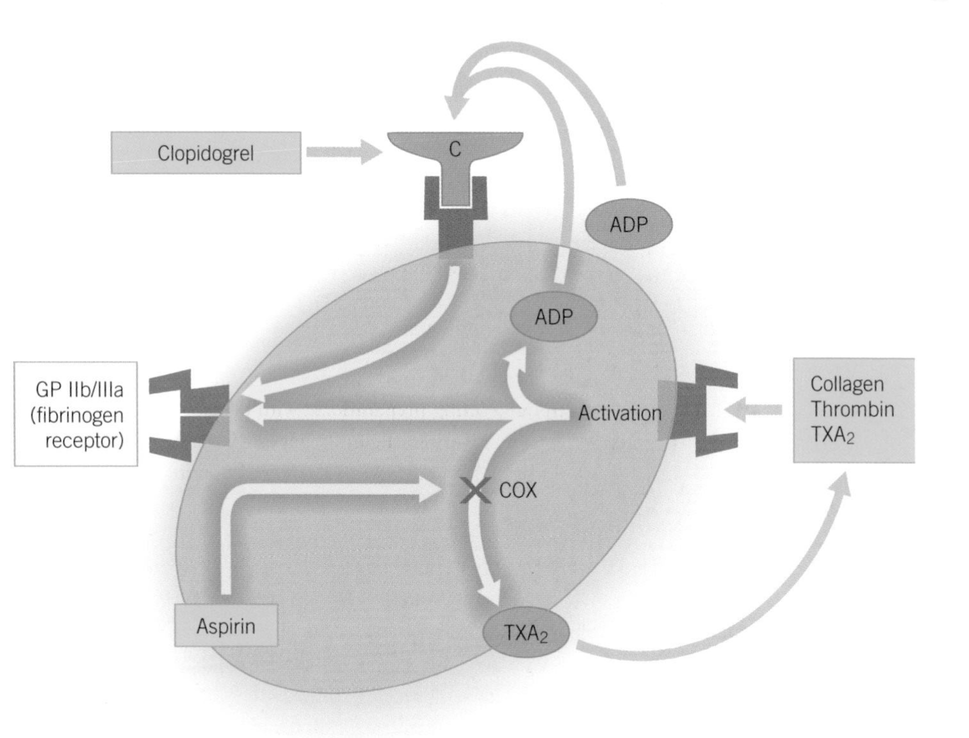

Fig. 34 Pathways resulting in platelet activation/aggregation. COX = cyclooxygenase; ADP = adenosine diphosphate; TXA_2 = thromboxane A_2; C = clopidogrel

threatening events. Aspirin should be administered as soon as possible after patient presentation of suspected ACS and continued indefinitely.[28] Aspirin exerts its effects primarily by interfering with the biosynthesis of cyclic prostanoids, i.e. thromboxane A_2 (TXA_2), prostacyclin, and other prostaglandins. These prostanoids are generated by the enzyme catalysed oxidation of arachidonic acid. The efficacy of aspirin has been clearly demonstrated in the Antithrombotic Trialists' Collaboration meta-analysis.[93] Its ability to prevent platelet aggregation appears to be its predominant mode of action. The absolute risk of vascular complications is the major determinant of the absolute benefit of antiplatelet prophylaxis (Figure 35).[94] High-risk patients derive the most benefit from aspirin, with a proportional risk reduction in serious vascular events of 46% in those with UA and 33% among those with stable angina.

Aspirin once daily is recommended in all clinical conditions in which antiplatelet prophylaxis has a favourable benefit/risk ratio.[95] The optimal dose of aspirin remains controversial, but available evidence supports the use of daily doses of aspirin in the range 75–100 mg (with 75 to 163 mg/day used in the US) for the long-term prevention of

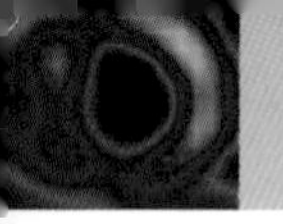

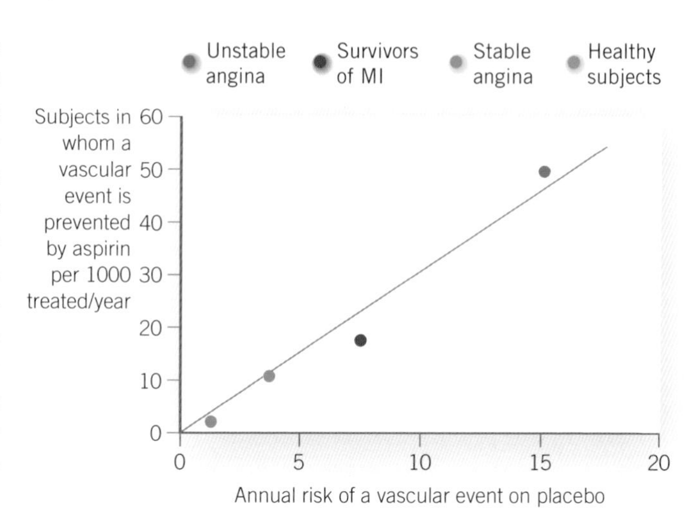

Fig. 35 Subjects in whom a vascular event is prevented by aspirin per 1000 treated/year versus annual risk of a vascular event on placebo. Reproduced with permission from Patrono C, Coller B, Dalen JE, et al. Platelet-Active Drugs: the relationship among dose, effectiveness, and side effects. Chest 1998;114:470S–488S. © American College of Chest Physicians

serious vascular events in high-risk patients (≥3% per year). Where an intermediate antithrombotic effect is required, e.g. an ACS, a loading dose of 160–300 mg (162–325 mg is the dose range recommended in the US)[96] should be given at diagnosis. Analysis of aspirin dose in the 12,526 subjects of the CURE study showed that medium-dose (101–199 mg/day) and high-dose (≥200 mg/day) aspirin had no advantage over low-dose (≤100 mg/day) aspirin whether patients receive combination therapy with clopidogrel or aspirin alone.[97] Furthermore, there was a significant 1.7 times increased bleeding rate with high- versus low-dose aspirin. In clinical practice most physicians in the US start with aspirin 325 mg since nearly 50% of cases will receive a stent. Thereafter using the CURE data the optimal aspirin dose is 75–100 mg/day.

“Aspirin is a mandatory treatment for ACS patients and it must be continued throughout life”

Due to the increase in the risk of upper gastrointestinal bleeding associated with aspirin use in the range 75–100 mg daily, it should not be used in individuals without ischaemic heart disease in whom any potential benefits of therapy are outweighed by the small risk of bleeding.

Up to a quarter of individuals may exhibit “aspirin resistance”, however no test of platelet function is recommended to assess the antiplatelet effect of aspirin in the individual patient as it is difficult to assess the clinical significance of *in vitro* platelet function studies.

Biochemical agonists play an important role in platelet activation and predominant agonists include: ADP, adrenaline (epinephrine), collagen, thrombin, serotonin, platelet activating factor (PAF) and TXA_2. It is estimated that there are over 100 such factors that might be involved in the process of platelet activation and subsequent thrombosis. Aspirin effectively inhibits the platelet aggregation response to collagen, ADP and thrombin (in low concentrations).

Although aspirin is the most widely prescribed agent to reduce coronary thrombosis, it has limitations; notably it is a relatively weak antiplatelet agent.[98] Thus aspirin may fail to provide full antithrombotic benefit. Aspirin therapy is also limited because it only blocks some of the stimuli that activate platelets leaving aspirin-independent pathways through which thrombosis can be precipitated.[99] A further potential problem is that ibuprofen interferes with the cardioprotective effects of aspirin and therefore it might be prudent to prescribe an alternative nonsteroidal anti-inflammatory drug (NSAID) in patients with, for example, chronic arthritis who are also taking low-dose aspirin for secondary prevention of cardiovascular disease.

“Higher-risk patients derive most benefits from aspirin treatment”

In patients with contraindications or who are intolerant to aspirin, or non-responders (aspirin failures), e.g. those who experience a cardiac event while taking aspirin, clopidogrel 75 mg daily is a suitable alternative.

Clopidogrel (Figure 36)

The CURE trial compared the benefit of aspirin plus clopidogrel (300 mg loading dose, then 75 mg/day) treatment versus aspirin alone in 12,562 patients with UA or NSTEMI treated for 3–12 months.[100] The use of clopidogrel reduced the risk of cardiovascular death, recurrent MI or stroke significantly by 20%. In addition there were similar

Fig. 36 Use of clopidogrel across the spectrum of ACS. DES = drug eluting stent.

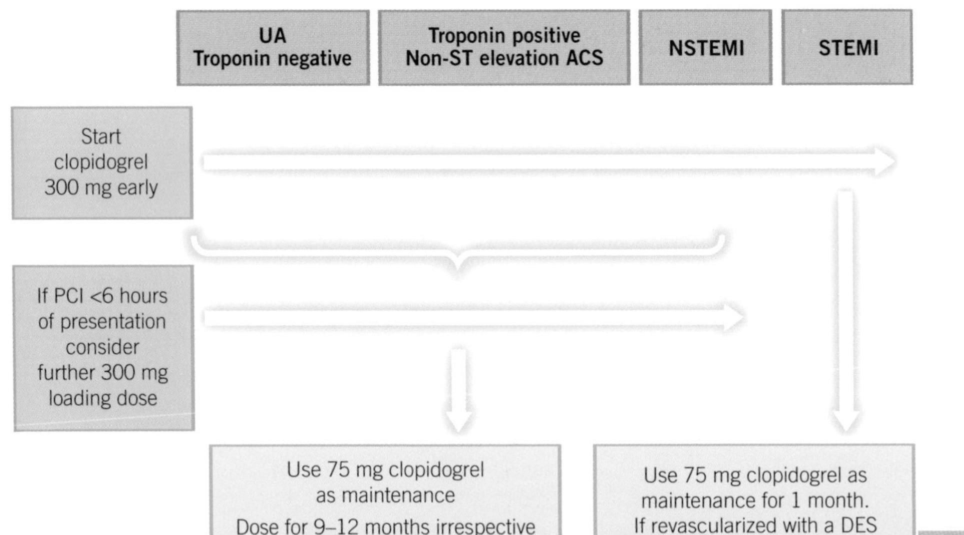

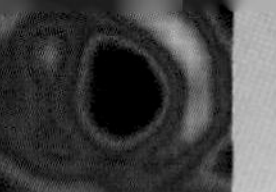

"In Europe start clopidogrel 300 mg at first contact and continue at a maintenance dose of 75 mg for 9–12 months"

"In the USA currently if CABG is not planned in the next 5 days or an early invasive strategy is planned withhold treatment until the coronary angiography is performed. In medically managed patients or where angiography will be delayed beyond 24-36 hours the guidelines are the same as in Europe"

"In Europe pretreat with 300 mg of clopidogrel for at least 6 hours and preferably 24 hours prior to PCI. If PCI is within 6 hours use a loading dose of 600 mg clopidogrel"

beneficial reductions in recurrent ischaemia with ECG changes resulting in rehospitalization or ischaemia leading to urgent revascularization. Clopidogrel was of benefit in the CURE trial irrespective of whether high-risk features were present, for example ECG changes or elevated cardiac biomarkers such as the cardiac troponins, suggesting a broad use for this agent as adjunctive therapy in all non-ST elevation ACS patients if no contraindication exists. The clinical benefit of clopidogrel in non-ST elevation ACS is rapid, appearing within 2 hours of initiation of therapy and is thus consistent with an early onset of action. The beneficial effects are not merely limited to this early phase, as analyses from CURE showed that the benefit in the first 30 days was similar to the benefit afforded after 30 days with ongoing treatment out to 1 year. Therefore patients should be started on treatment early and treatment should be continued beyond the acute phase.

Adjunctive therapy for PCI

PCI-CURE was a substudy of the CURE trial that evaluated the benefit of pretreatment and long-term therapy with clopidogrel in 2658 ACS patients prior to PCI.[101] Every patient received open-label thienopyridine after PCI for approximately 30 days, following which blinded original study drug was restarted for a further 8 months. On average, patients were pretreated for 6–10 days prior to PCI. Pretreatment with clopidogrel reduced the risk of cardiovascular death, recurrent MI or target vessel revascularization within 30 days of PCI by 30%. Interestingly the prior use of clopidogrel reduced the need for GP IIb/IIIa inhibitors at angiography. Similarly long-term treatment (on average for 9 months) was associated with a reduction in cardiovascular risk compared with those who merely received clopidogrel for 1 month following PCI. The benefits of pretreatment and long-term therapy with clopidogrel prior to PCI were also observed in the CREDO trial.[102] CREDO investigated pretreatment with clopidogrel 300 mg followed by 75 mg maintenance therapy in a population of ACS and elective patients treated for 1 year. Patients allocated to placebo received clopidogrel for 1 month after PCI and placebo thereafter. The benefit of pretreatment was observed only among those who had pretreatment more than 6 hours prior to PCI. Taken together the PCI-CURE and CREDO trials suggest that ACS patients should be treated early with clopidogrel prior to PCI and treatment continued long term for 9–12 months.

Initiation of therapy and loading dose

Most patients with non-ST elevation ACS are admitted to non-specialist centres with perhaps little facility for emergency cardiac

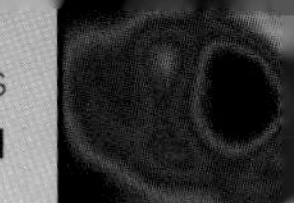

catheterization available on site. Such patients undergo cardiac catheterization often after a minimum delay of 24 hours. While the ACC/AHA[28,103] and the American College of Chest Physicians (ACCP)[104] recommend withholding clopidogrel until it is known whether a patient will undergo bypass surgery within the next few days, the developments in PCI mean that today most patients are

Fig. 37
Recommendations of the ACC/AHA, ACCP and ESC for the use of clopidogrel in non-ST elevation ACS.[28,104–106]

	ACC/AHA 2002	ACCP 2004	ESC guidelines 2005
Recommendations in non-ST elevation ACS	In patients in whom an early non-interventional approach is planned administer clopidogrel 300 mg to all patients if no contraindication exists as early as possible followed by 75 mg for 1–9 months	In all patients in whom diagnostic cardiac catheterization will be delayed or if CABG will occur in >5 days, clopidogrel 300 mg followed by 75 mg for 9–12 months is recommended	Administer clopidogrel 300 mg to all patients if no contraindication exists at first contact followed by 75 mg for 9–12 months
	In patients who have angiography within <24–36hours, it is recommended that clopidogrel be initially withheld and given after the coronary anatomy is identified if CABG is not planned in the next 5 days	In patients who have angiography within 24 hours, it is recommended that clopidogrel be initially withheld and given after the coronary anatomy is identified if CABG is not planned in the next 5 days	
Level of recommendation	IB	IA	IB
Recommendations for clopidogrel loading in patients undergoing PCI	NA	Clopidogrel may be administered after PCI. The recommendations are to use 300 mg loading dose; an alternative higher dose of 600 mg could also be considered (lower evidence base)	Pretreat preferably for 24 hours with clopidogrel 300 mg. If PCI within <6 hours of presentation pretreat with 600 mg. If pretreatment not possible treat with 600 mg as early as possible
Level of recommendation	NA	IB, 2C	IC

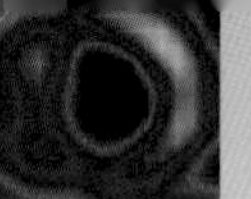

revascularized percutaneously (Figure 37). The observation that patients gain benefit even a few hours after initiation of dual antiplatelet therapy with clopidogrel and aspirin has led the ESC to issue guidelines[105] recommending the immediate use of clopidogrel 300 mg for the management of non-ST elevation ACS (Figure 37). In patients undergoing PCI it is recommended that this dose be given at least 6 hours prior to PCI. If PCI is planned within 2 hours then 600 mg clopidogrel should be administered. Thus in tertiary centres patients pretreated with clopidogrel for more than 6 hours will not routinely be given any additional loading dose prior to cardiac catheterization. If the patient requires a coronary artery bypass graft (CABG) clopidogrel will usually be withheld for 5 days prior to surgery and restarted thereafter. The ESC guidelines reinforce the trial data and recommend that patients with non-ST elevation ACS should be continued on clopidogrel for 9–12 months irrespective of whether they undergo PCI. Irrespective of clinical presentation, patients who receive a drug-eluting stent should continue clopidogrel for 12 months.

“In the USA clopidogrel can be given at the end of PCI. The loading dose of 300 mg is generally recommended but the 600 mg dose is at physician's discretion”

“Whatever the clinical presentation, patients receiving drug-eluting stents as part of percutaneous revascularization should be given clopidogrel 75 mg maintenance for 1 year”

Safety

While overall the use of clopidogrel is associated with a slightly higher rate of bleeding in non-ST elevation ACS, there appears to be no excess in major bleeding after bypass both in STEMI and in non-ST elevation ACS patients. In particular there is no increase in haemorrhagic strokes. The risk of bleeding increases with the dose of concomitant aspirin used and so the optimum dose of long-term aspirin is 75–100 mg following ACS when used with clopidogrel 75 mg daily. Unlike ticlopidine, the first major drug of this class, the use of clopidogrel does not require regular monitoring to screen for neutropenia.

Newer agents

While clopidogrel is a highly effective treatment for all patients with ACS a number of potential limitations remain. First, clopidogrel results in irreversible platelet inhibition and therefore needs to be discontinued 5 days prior to surgery. In addition approximately 25% of patients appear to be resistant to clopidogrel as assessed by platelet aggregometry and this in turn may be associated with worse cardio-vascular outcomes.[107] This, coupled with a need for a drug with a faster onset of action, has led to newer third generation drugs such as prasugrel, cangrelor and AZD1640.[108] Prasugrel, like clopidogrel, binds irreversibly to the ADP P_2Y_{12} receptor and is currently being compared against clopidogrel in ACS patients undergoing PCI in a

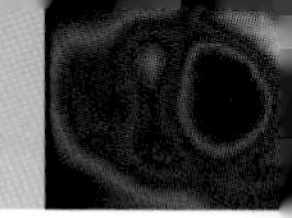

phase III trial. The clinical data to date suggest that prasugrel may not have the same problem of resistance as clopidogrel due to conversion of the pro-drug to the active metabolite in the blood stream. Cangrelor and AZD1640 are competitive antagonists of the P_2Y_{12} receptor, which therefore have the advantage of a fast onset of action. However, as the duration of benefit is the half-life of the drug rather than the life span of the platelet, use of these drugs would not delay bypass surgery. The safety of these agents in ACS patients is currently being assessed.

Intravenous antiplatelet therapies

GP IIb/IIIa receptor inhibitors

Circulating platelets play a critical role in normal haemostatic function, however platelet aggregation and thrombosis are maladaptive processes in ACS and contribute to ischaemic complications of PCI. Atherosclerotic plaque rupture during ACS and PCI exposes thrombogenic subendothelial components leading to platelet deposition and activation.[109] Platelet activation is associated with surface expression of greater numbers of GP IIb/IIIa receptors available for binding fibrin strands and platelet cross-linking. In addition to cross-linking as part of the aggregation process, activated platelets release local mediators that can induce further platelet accumulation and activation, vasoconstriction, thrombosis and mitogenesis. Platelet activation leads not only to thrombus formation in epicardial artery arteries, but also distal embolization and plugging of the microcirculation, which have been associated with poor outcomes.[110,111]

“Unlike abciximab, eptifibatide and tirofiban, the two small-molecule agents, may be started 1 or 2 days before, and continued during PCI for medically treated only (not PCI) patients”

Several large randomized clinical trials have demonstrated improved clinical outcomes associated with the administration of GP IIb/IIIa receptor antagonists among patients presenting with ACS and after PCI.[112] While iv agents appear to be beneficial, the oral GP IIb/IIIa inhibitors, in contrast, have been ineffective and may increase mortality. Three iv GP IIb/IIIa inhibitors are currently available for clinical use: abciximab, tirofiban and eptifibatide. Abciximab is a GP IIb/IIIa inhibitor comprised of the Fab fragment of the chimeric human-murine monoclonal antibody 7E3. Tirofiban is a nonpeptide inhibitor of the platelet GP IIb/IIIa receptor, interfering with aggregation by mimicking the geometric, stereotactic, and charge characteristics of the platelet integrin-binding domain sequence. Eptifibatide is a non-immunogenic, cyclic heptapeptide with an active pharmacophore that is derived from the structure of barbourin, a platelet GP IIb/IIIa inhibitor from the venom of the Southeastern pigmy rattlesnake.[113] The US Food and Drug Administration (FDA)-approved indications for use of these medications in the management of CAD are shown in Figure 38.

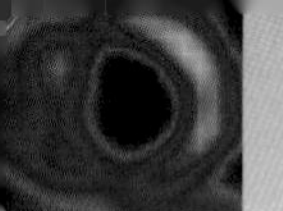

Fig. 38 FDA-approved indications for the use of GP IIb/IIIa inhibitors in CAD.

Indication	Eptifibatide*	Abciximab	Tirofiban^
UA/NSTEMI medically managed	180 g/kg followed by 2.0 g/kg/min until hospital discharge or CABG, up to 72 hours[114]	Contraindicated Death at 48 hours was 0.3% (placebo), 0.7% (abciximab for 24 hours), and 0.9% (abciximab for 48 hours, p=0.008 versus placebo)[118]	0.4 g/kg/min administered for 30 minutes followed by 0.1 g/kg/min for 48 to 108 hours[116,117] (PRISM-PLUS dose)
UA/NSTEMI with PCI	180 g/kg and a second 180 g/kg bolus 10 minutes later followed by intravenous infusion of 2.0 g/kg/min for 18–24 hours after angiography[122]	0.25 mg/kg administered over 10–60 minutes before the start of PCI, followed by intravenous infusion of 0.125 g/kg/min (to a maximum of 10 g/min) for 12 hours[128]	10 g/kg followed by infusion of 0.15 g/kg/min for 18 to 24 hours[115]

* Patients with an estimated clearance (using the Cockroft-Gault equation) 50 mL/min or, if creatinine clearance is not available, a serum creatinine >2.0 mg/dL should receive half the usual rate of infusion

^ Patients with an estimated clearance (using the Cockroft-Gault equation) 30 mL/min should receive half the usual rate of infusion

GP IIb/IIIa inhibition in medically treated patients with UA/NSTEMI

Among UA/NSTEMI patients treated with medical therapy alone, benefit has been demonstrated with eptifibatide (PURSUIT)[114] and tirofiban (RESTORE, PRISM and PRISM-PLUS).[115–117] In contrast mortality was higher among medically only treated patients who received abciximab in the GUSTO-IV–ACS trial.[118]

A meta-analysis of GP IIb/IIIa antagonists in six large trials involving 31,402 UA/NSTEMI patients who were not scheduled to undergo PCI was conducted by Boersma *et al.*[119] Significant reduction in the odds for the combined endpoint of death or MI was observed in the GP IIb/IIIa antagonist group at 5 days (5.7% versus 6.9% for placebo/control, odds ratio [OR] 0.84, 95% confidence interval [CI] 0.77 to 0.93) and at 30 days (10.8% versus 11.8%, OR 0.91, 95% CI 0.85–0.98). Bleeding was increased significantly (2.4% versus 1.4%, $p<0.0001$) but no increase in intracranial bleeding (0.09% versus 0.06%) was noted. The observed benefit of GP IIb/IIIa antagonists however, was largely confined to patients who went on to have PCI or CABG within 30 days (OR for death or MI 0.89, 95% CI 0.80–0.98). For those

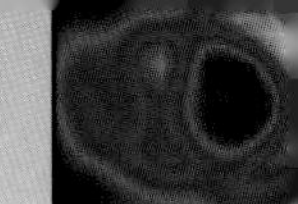

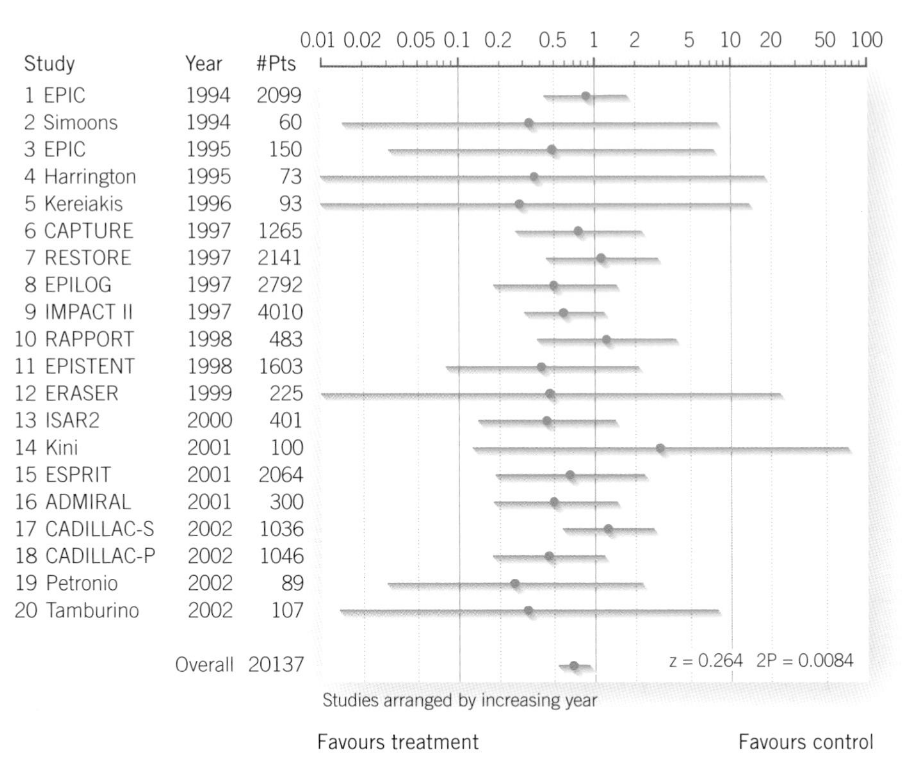

Fig. 39 Mortality at 30 days. Meta-analysis of 19 randomized, placebo-controlled trials of GP IIb/IIIa receptor antagonists (20 comparisons, n=20,137) demonstrating a significant reduction in mortality at 30 days (RR 0.69; 95% CI 0.53 to 0.90). Reproduced with permission from Karvouni E, Katritsis DG, Ioannidis JPA. Intravenous glycoprotein IIb/IIIa receptor antagonists reduce mortality after percutaneous coronary interventions. J Am Coll Cardiol 2003;41:26–32. © Elsevier

patients, 25,555 (81%) in this analysis, who did *not* undergo early revascularization there was no significant reduction in death or MI (OR 0.95, 95% CI 0.86–1.05). The benefit of therapy also appeared to be limited to patients with a positive TnT or TnI concentration (0.1 ng/mL) (OR 0.85, 95% CI 0.71–1.03). In a subsequent meta-analysis, Karvouni *et al.* demonstrated over a 30% reduction in mortality with GP IIb/IIIa inhibitors (Figure 39).[120] The benefit was largely confined to eptifibatide and abciximab, and not tirofiban. A test of heterogeneity showed that the mortality was no different for eptifibatide and abciximab.

“Use any GP IIb/IIIa antagonist for patients who will have PCI”

GP IIb/IIIa inhibition in routine PCI patients and patients with UA/NSTEMI treated with PCI

GP IIb/IIIa antagonists have been shown to reduce ischaemic complications of routine PCI and are indicated during routine procedures.[121–123] Few PCI trials have directly compared the efficacy of

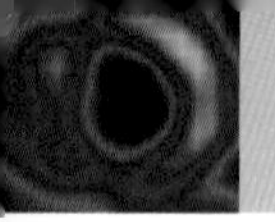

abciximab, tirofiban, and eptifibatide.[124] The efficacy of abciximab and tirofiban was assessed in the TARGET trial (n=4809).[123] Abciximab was superior to tirofiban in the reduction of death, infarction, or the need for urgent revascularization at 30 days (6% versus 7.6%, hazard ratio 0.79). The benefit was mainly limited to patients undergoing stent implantation for ACS. There was no significant difference by 6 months of follow-up between the two agents.[125] The initial benefit with abciximab compared with tirofiban may have been due to greater levels of platelet inhibition with abciximab versus tirofiban, but a higher dose of tirofiban was evaluated in the STRATEGY trial of STEMI patients undergoing primary PCI and no difference in death or recurrent MI were observed between abciximab and tirofiban.[126]

“GP IIb/IIIa antagonists are most beneficial in patients with positive cardiac biomarkers, and those who undergo PCI”

All three GP IIb/IIIa receptor antagonists have been shown to reduce the incidence of death or MI in patients with UA/NSTEMI undergoing PCI.[103,114,117,127,128] An analysis of data from 12,296 patients in CAPTURE, PURSUIT, and PRISM-PLUS using abciximab, eptifibatide and tirofiban, respectively, demonstrated that iv GP IIb/IIIa inhibition added to heparin and aspirin significantly reduced the rate of death or non-fatal MI during drug infusion (2.5% versus 3.8%) and during the first 48 hours after PCI (4.9% versus 8%).[129] The benefit from GP IIb/IIIa inhibition was primarily observed among troponin positive patients.[130,131] Data from over 60,000 patients in the NRMI registry demonstrate a 5.5% absolute reduction in mortality when GP IIb/IIIa inhibition is initiated within the first 24 hours. In a multivariate model, and after adjustment for the propensity to be treated with such agents, there was a significant 12% relative risk reduction.[132] Tirofiban and eptifibatide are substantially less expensive than abciximab and their use is associated with lower hospital and 30-day costs.

“Intravenous UFH is key in the management of all UA/NSTEMI ACS patients”

Antithrombin therapy

ACS are precipitated by rupture of a vulnerable atherosclerotic plaque superimposed with thrombus that completely or partially occludes the culprit artery. The generation of thrombin is key to forming fibrin strands, activating platelets and ultimately creating a stable clot. Antithrombotic agents, such as unfractionated heparin (UFH), LMWH and direct thrombin inhibitors, target this critical step.[133]

Unfractionated heparin

UFH reduces thrombin generation and activity. Its effects are mediated by a cofactor, antithrombin, which inactivates fluid-phase factor IIa (thrombin), factor IXa, and factor X. This underlies the rationale for its use in ACS.[133]

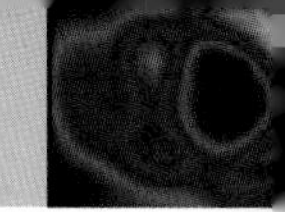

Unfractionated heparin	Class**
• IV UFH or subcutaneous LMWH should be added to antiplatelet therapy	I
Low molecular weight heparin	
• IV UFH or subcutaneous LMWH should be added to antiplatelet therapy	I
• Enoxaparin is preferable to UFH as an anticoagulant unless CABG is planned within 24 hours	IIa
Direct thrombin inhibitors	
• Hirudin may be an acceptable alternative to UFH in patients with heparin-induced thrombocytopenia	–
• Bivalirudin may be used as an anticoagulant in UA patients undergoing PCI	–

** Evidence classified as per the ACC/AHA Task Force on Practice Guidelines:[133]

Class I: Evidence and/or agreement that a given procedure is useful, beneficial, and effective

Class II: Conflicting evidence and/or a divergence of opinion about the usefulness/efficacy of a procedure or treatment: a) weight of evidence/opinion favours usefulness/efficacy; b) usefulness/efficacy less well established by evidence/opinion

Class III: Evidence and/or agreement that a procedure/treatment is not useful/effective and in some cases may be harmful

Fig. 40
Recommendations for antithrombotic use in UA/NSTEMI. As per the ACC/AHA Task Force on Practice Guidelines;[133] no significant differences with the ESC guidelines.

Clinical experience

In UA, iv UFH significantly reduced the risk of MI and recurrent refractory angina by 89% and 63% respectively.[133,134] In a head-to-head comparison rates of MI were lower with UFH than aspirin (0.8% versus 3.7%, p=0.035).[135] The greatest benefits appeared during UFH therapy, with an important risk of rebound ischaemia when the drug was stopped.[136] A meta-analysis of six UA trials showed a 33% (p=0.06) reduction in the risk of death or MI at 2–12 weeks among patients treated with both heparin and aspirin versus aspirin alone.[137]

Among UA/NSTEMI patients aspirin reduced the risk of death and MI in the RISC trial.[138] Although patients treated with UFH alone showed no benefit, those who received both heparin and aspirin had the fewest events during the first 5 days. A meta-analysis of four UA/NSTEMI trials further supports combination therapy, with a significant reduction in the risk of death or MI during the first week by 54% (p=0.016) in patients treated with heparin and aspirin versus aspirin alone.[133] Importantly the administration of UFH with aspirin appears to reduce ischaemic complications by attenuating the reactivation of the primary disease process.[133]

“The pharmacokinetic profile of UFH varies requiring frequent monitoring of anticoagulant levels”

"Thrombocytopenia and HIT are important potential side effects"

Recommendations and dosing

UFH in addition to antiplatelet drugs are the cornerstones of therapy in UA/NSTEMI and are accepted by both the ACC/AHA and the ESC (Figure 40).[35,133] A weight-based UFH regimen is preferable with a bolus of 60 to 70 U/kg (maximum 5000 U) followed by an infusion of 12 to 15 U/kg/hour (maximum 1000 U) for 2 to 5 days. The activated partial thromboplastin time (aPTT) is frequently monitored (every 6 hours after dose adjustments to a target aPTT at 1.5 to 2.5 times control, then daily thereafter). Daily platelet and haemoglobin/haematocrit measurements are also recommended.[133]

Limitations

UFH is a mixture of polypeptide chains of varying length with important pharmacokinetic consequences. UFH binds to many plasma proteins resulting in poor bioavailability. The anticoagulant response is variable among patients. For example, higher doses may be required in diabetics, smokers and patients weighing over 100 kg while lower doses may be adequate in elderly women. Monitoring anticoagulation levels accurately is difficult since therapeutic ranges for aPTT are not standardized between laboratories. In addition platelet counts need to be followed for the development of mild or severe thrombocytopenia in 10–20% and 1–2% of patients respectively, usually following 4–14 days of UFH therapy.[133] Rarely, autoimmune heparin-induced thrombocytopenia (HIT) may occur with dangerous prothrombotic risks and should be investigated when platelet counts drop to <100,000.[139] These limitations have encouraged the development of alternative antithrombin drugs.

"Subcutaneous enoxaparin, a LMWH, is superior to UFH in UA/NSTEMI ACS in reducing ischaemic complications, with the additional advantages of a more stable pharmacokinetic profile, no aPTT monitoring and less thrombocytopenia"

Low molecular weight heparins

LMWHs are prepared by depolymerization of UFH into shorter peptides of lower weight (5000 Da) containing a pentasaccharide unit key for the binding of antithrombin and inhibiting factor Xa.[140] The advantages of LMWH over UFH include increased anti-Xa:anti-IIa activity with more effective inhibition of thrombin generation and less binding to plasma proteins resulting in a stable long-acting systemic anticoagulant effect that does not require aPTT monitoring. There is greater resistance to platelet factor IV and activated platelets with less thrombocytopenia and HIT.[57,140]

Clinical experience

LMWH has been well studied in UA/NSTEMI ACS. Dalteparin reduced death/MI through day 6 by 63% among aspirin-treated patients in the FRISC study compared with placebo.[133] Trials

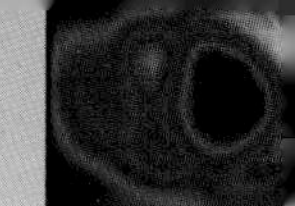

testing the superiority of dalteparin (the FRIC trial) and fraxiparine (the FRAXIS trial) versus UFH were disappointing and may be partly explained by the reduced anti-Xa:anti-IIa activity of these LMWHs compared with others, such as enoxaparin.[140] In support of this ESSENCE and TIMI IIB both demonstrated *superiority* with enoxaparin, a LMWH with high anti-Xa:anti-IIa activity (3.8:1), compared with UFH in reducing cardiovascular events by 20%.[133,140] Importantly treatment benefits with enoxaparin were observed early (within 48 hours) applied to patients treated conservatively or invasively and were present even when compared with patients who achieved appropriate anticoagulation levels with UFH.[140]

Recently enoxaparin versus UFH has been investigated with GP IIb/IIIa inhibitors. In the INTERACT trial there was significantly less non-CABG major bleeding and death/MI with enoxaparin. Importantly revascularization procedures were *delayed* (median time 101 hours).[141] A to Z showed a trend to improved cardiac events by 11%, significant among the subgroup managed *conservatively*.[142] However in SYNERGY, a trial of *early* invasive management with platelet GP IIb/IIIa inhibitors, enoxaparin was non-inferior to UFH for death/MI by day 30 but was associated with increased TIMI major bleeding.[143] These data suggest that enoxaparin is safest and beneficial among UA/NSTEMI patients on GP IIb/IIIa inhibitors managed with a *conservative* or *delayed* invasive approach; UFH is preferable for an *early* invasive strategy.

> *“LMWH should not be used in patients over 75 years or with significant renal dysfunction”*

Recommendations and dosing

Enoxaparin is accepted as an anticoagulant in UA/NSTEMI (Figure 40).[35,133] Twice daily subcutaneous administration (1 mg/kg) achieves appropriate anticoagulation levels without the need for aPTT monitoring.[57] Although associated with less thrombocytopenia,[140] platelet counts should be measured. Based on data from STEMI clinical trials it is prudent not to use LMWH in patients with significant renal dysfunction or in the elderly (i.e. >75 years).[139] Among patients undergoing PCI enoxaparin should be held on the morning of the procedure and, if more than 8 hours elapses from the last dose, UFH should be started. If coronary artery bypass is planned UFH is preferable to LMWH since its anticoagulant effects are more readily reversed with protamine.[133]

> *“Hirudin is an alternative to UFH among UA/NSTEMI ACS patients with HIT”*

Direct thrombin inhibitors

Direct thrombin inhibitors, such as hirudin and bivalirudin, are theoretically advantageous to UFH because they:

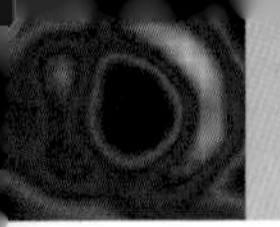

1. Bind directly and tightly with thrombin without the need for co-factors such as antithrombin III.
2. Are more effective in inhibiting fluid-phase and clot-bound thrombin.
3. Do not cause or aggravate HIT.
4. Achieve more stable levels of anticoagulation.[140]

> *"Bivalirudin may be used as an anticoagulant in UA patients for PCI instead of UFH"*

Clinical experience

Hirudin has shown limited or no additional clinical effects in UA/NSTEMI patients compared with UFH. In GUSTO-IIb the risk of death/MI at 30 days with hirudin versus UFH was similar among UA/NSTEMI patients.[144] In OASIS-2, a much larger trial, there was a *trend* to improvement in death/MI by 7 days with hirudin over UFH but major bleeding, though uncommon, was increased.[145] However in a meta-analysis of all hirudin ACS trials (UA/NSTEMI and STEMI) there was a 10% benefit ($p=0.02$) with hirudin over UFH in reducing death/MI by day 35.[133]

Recently bivalirudin with provisional GP IIb/IIIa inhibition has been shown to be non-inferior to UFH with GP IIb/IIIa inhibition among patients undergoing PCI in REPLACE-2 with similar reductions in ischaemic complications but *significantly less* in-hospital major bleeding (2.4% versus 4.1%, $p<0.001$).[146] However only 14% of patients had UA within 48 hours prior to PCI, highlighting the need for further research to define the role of bivalirudin in UA/NSTEMI.

> *"When possible, an early invasive strategy is preferred for medium- to high-risk patients"*

Recommendations and dosing

Hirudin can be used as an alternative to heparin among patients with HIT in UA/NSTEMI[35,133] and is administered as a bolus (0.4 mg/kg iv over 15 to 20 seconds) followed by an iv infusion (0.15 mg/kg/hour) targeted to 1.5 to 2.5 times control aPTT values (Figure 40).[133]

In the US and most of Europe, bivalirudin is approved for anticoagulation in patients with UA undergoing PCI.[139] The dosing regimen in REPLACE-2 was a bolus of bivalirudin of 0.75 mg/kg prior to PCI, then 1.75 mg/kg/hour for the duration of the procedure.[146]

Factor Xa inhibitor

The heparin binding site consists of five sugar molecules which allow heparin to bind antithrombin inducing a conformational change, increasing the ability of antithrombin to inactivate thrombin and factors Xa, XIa, IXa. Synthetic pentasaccharides have been created to mimic the effects of heparin and alter the inhibitory profile. Fondaparinux is the first of these to be extensively studied. When

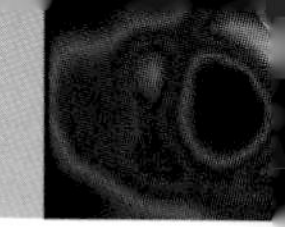

fondaparinux binds to antithrombin it provides a very specific inhibition of factor Xa without interfering with other clotting factors.

The OASIS 5 trial[147] compared fondaparinux 2.5 mg once daily with enoxaparin 1 mg/kg twice daily in 20,078 UA/NSTEMI patients in addition to standard treatment (aspirin, clopidogrel and GP IIb/IIIa inhibitors). At 9 days there was no significant difference between the two treatment arms for the combined endpoint of death, MI, or refractory ischaemia. However there was a significant reduction in total bleeding, major bleeding, minor bleeding and the need for blood transfusions in the fondaparinux group compared with those receiving enoxaparin ($p<0.0001$). At 6 months fondaparinux was associated with a significant reduction in mortality compared with enoxaparin (10.3% versus 11.2%, $p=0.04$). It is possible that these results represent better dosing of fondaparinux rather than intrinsic differences in the properties of these two drugs, however, until trials address this issue, fondaparinux would appear preferable to enoxaparin in the treatment of ACS.

"Fondaparinux would appear preferable to enoxaparin in the treatment of ACS"

Medical versus surgical revascularization

PCI and CABG

The benefits of routine invasive versus selective invasive approaches to UA/NSTEMI remain controversial. The ACC/AHA Practice Guidelines include both an early invasive and early conservative strategy. Unstable patients with recurrent chest pain/ischaemia, heart failure or serious arrhythmias should be sent for early angiography. Stable patients can undergo non-invasive risk stratification using stress testing to select medical or invasive treatment. Many clinicians however question the accuracy of this ischaemia-driven non-invasive risk approach and advocate anatomy-driven stratification based on coronary angiography. Additionally advances in PCI, especially with the use of intracoronary stents, has shifted many physicians to adopt the strategy of urgent primary angioplasty.

Early invasive and conservative strategies were compared in the TIMI IIIB trial.[148] Results showed no difference between either group in the incidence of death or non-fatal MI after 1 year. Similarly the VANQWISH trial[149] showed that most patients with non-Q-wave MI did not benefit from routine early invasive management. These early trials were limited by not having the added benefits of intracoronary stents and adjunctive medical therapies with GP IIb/IIIa receptor blockers, LMWHs, and thienopyridines. Subsequent randomized clinical trials in which stents were commonly employed have shown that an early invasive approach with cardiac catheterization is superior

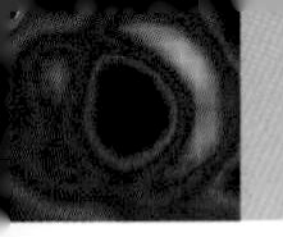

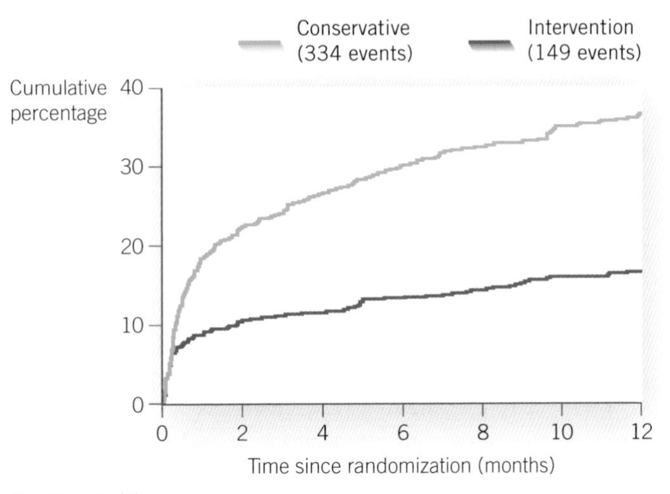

Number at risk

Intervention	895	787	720
Conservative	915	666	555

Fig. 41 Intervention halved the likelihood of death, MI, refractory angina or further revascularization. The frequency of refractory angina in the conservative group was significantly greater than in the intervention group at 4 months and at 1 year. Reproduced with permission from Fox KAA, Poole-Wilson PA, Henderson RA, et al; Randomized Intervention Trial of unstable Angina Investigators. Interventional versus conservative treatment for patients with unstable angina or non-ST-elevation myocardial infarction: The British Heart Foundation RITA 3 randomised trial. Lancet 2002;360:743–751. http://image.thelancet.com/extras/02art8090web.pdf © Elsevier

"All patients should receive aggressive pharmacologic therapy including: aspirin, clopidogrel, UFH or LMWH (enoxaparin preferred), and anti-ischaemic medications (beta-blockers, glyceryl trinitrate)"

to an initial conservative approach that reserves coronary angiography for patients who develop recurrent ischaemia despite initial medical therapy. Both FRISC-II[150] and TACTICS-TIMI-18[151] demonstrated significant reduction of death, recurrent MI and hospitalization using the invasive approach. In FRISC-II the 1-year mortality in the invasive strategy group was 2.2% versus 3.9% in the non-invasive strategy group (p=0.016). In TACTICS-TIMI-18 death or MI at 6 months was 7.3% in the invasive group compared with 9.5% in the non-invasive group (p<0.05). The addition of a GP IIb/IIa inhibitor probably added to the better outcome in the early invasive treated patients. Clinical benefit was primarily seen in patients in the higher-risk NSTEMI group identified by elevated troponins. The RITA-3 study performed in the UK[152] revealed a 50% reduction of refractory angina with the interventional approach (Figure 41). Death and MI were similar for both strategies at 1 year, but only 18% of patients in this study had elevated biomarkers. Based on these data the

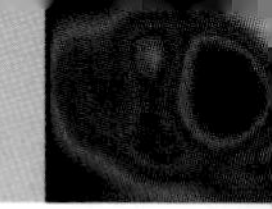

ACC/AHA practice guidelines for the management of UA/NSTEMI were revised in 2002 assigning early invasive management of UA/NSTEMI a Class I (level of evidence: A) recommendation for patients with moderate to high risk.[28] Moderate to high risk is defined as one or more of the following:

- high TIMI risk score
- rest or low-level exercise ischaemia despite medical therapy
- elevated troponins
- new ST depression
- congestive heart failure (CHF)
- prior revascularization
- haemodynamic or electrical instability.

“GP IIb/IIIa receptor antagonists provide added benefit for moderate- to high-risk patients”

For low-risk patients the ACC/AHA guidelines suggest either an early non-invasive or early invasive approach (Class I indication, evidence B). Risk stratification of ACS (see pages 32–35) should start with an ECG and measurement of troponins. UA (biomarker negative) patients can be further risk stratified using non-invasive stress testing whereas NSTEMI (biomarker positive) patients appear to benefit by early catheterization. However the ICTUS investigators[153] found that there was no advantage in early intervention among NSTEMI patients with elevated troponins who were given optimized medical therapy. ISAR-COOL,[154] a trial with tirofiban, demonstrated that delaying catheterization to let medication “stabilize” the vessel did *not* improve outcome, but rather it was associated with higher adverse events.

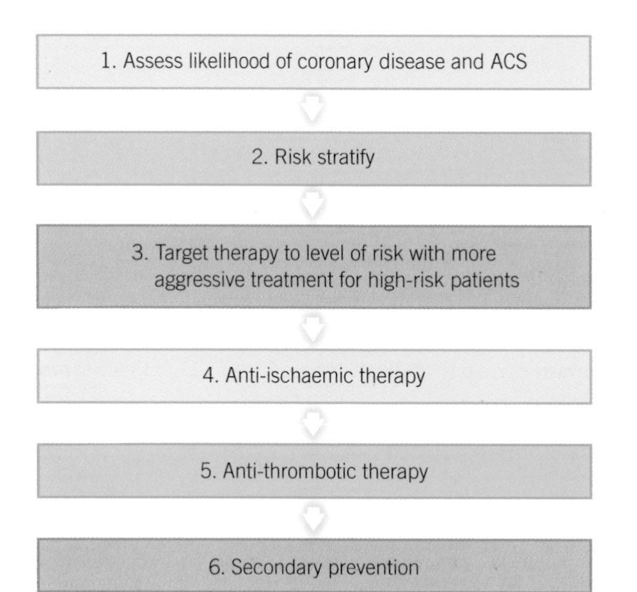

Fig. 42 Overview of management of NSTEMI.

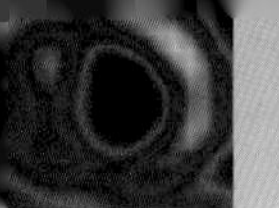

Summary guidelines

Findings from the GRACE registry, which records data from 95 hospitals in 14 countries worldwide, shows that the substantial differences in management of UA/NSTEMI are based on hospital type and geographical location. The impact of such differences on subsequent survival is now being studied but presently GRACE provides a reference standard for the uptake of therapies of proven efficacy.

Algorithms for medical and invasive treatment of UA/NSTEMI should be based on:

1. Type of ACS (UA or NSTEMI)
2. Risk catagorization (TIMI risk score)
3. Geographic site-of-care.

Fig. 43 Emergency checklist for the management of NSTEMI.

1. Assessment	a. Chest pain status b. TIMI risk score
2. Initial testing	a. ECG b. CK-MB and troponin Q8H x2 c. Chest X-ray
3. Medications	a. Aspirin b. Oxygen c. Clopidogrel d. GP IIb/IIIa (high risk) e. LMWH or UFH f. Nitrates g. Beta-blocker

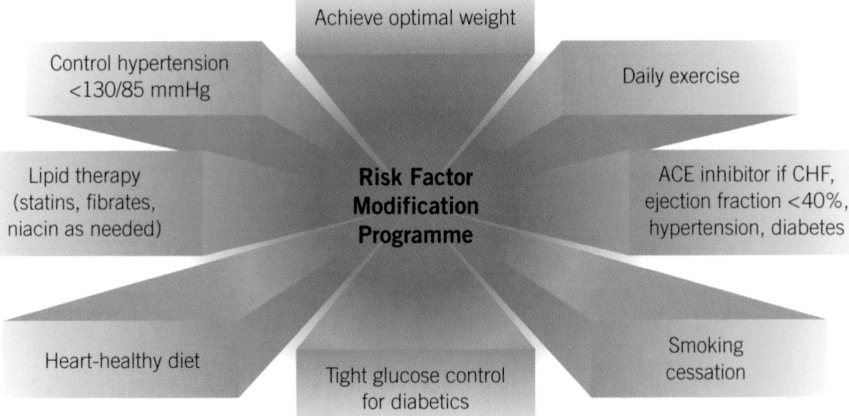

Fig. 44 Risk factor modification programme.

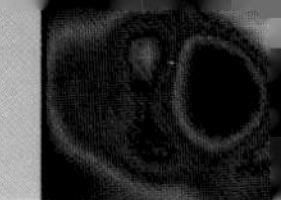

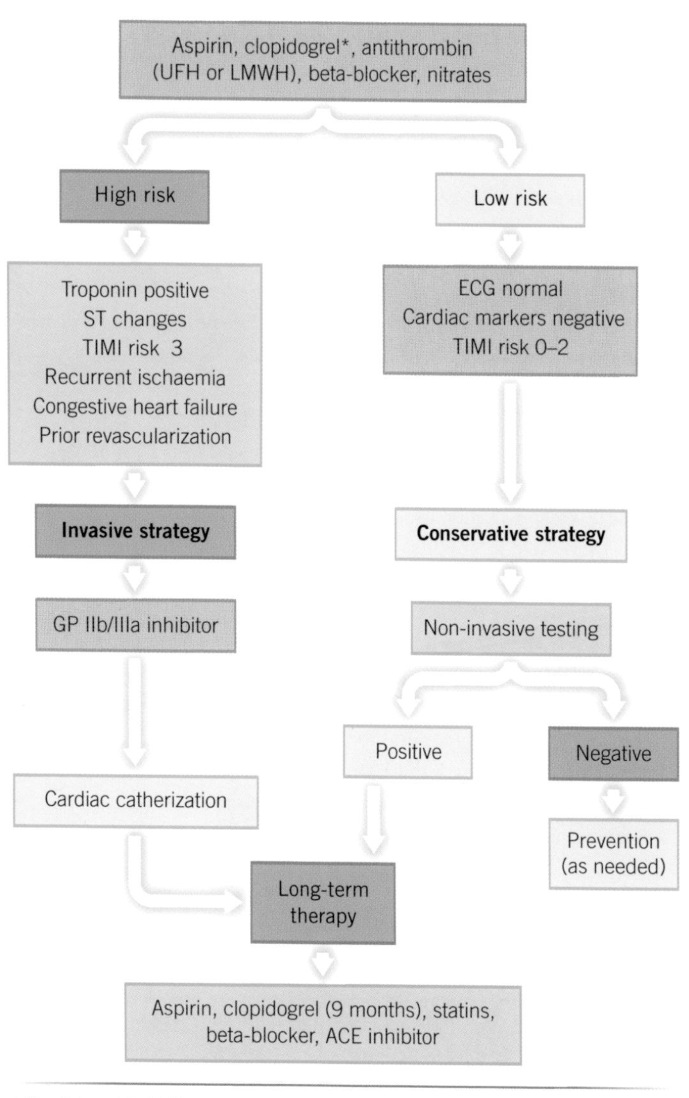

*Clopidogrel held if likely cardiac surgery

Fig. 45 Summary of treatment strategies in NSTEMI.

Site-of-care considerations are distinguished by a hospital *with* the availability of on-site interventional catheterization and CABG versus a hospital *without* PCI or CABG. Outlined here are a general overview (Figure 42), emergency checklist (Figure 43), a risk factor modification programme (Figure 44), and summary treatment strategies (Figure 45).

Management of STEMI

General treatment guidelines

Guidelines for the management of STEMI have been recently updated by the ACC, AHA and the Canadian Cardiovascular Society.[155] The following discussion summarizes many of the recommendations put forth in these practice recommendations.

Pathophysiology

“Risk stratification into low-, medium-, and high-risk group aids treatment planning”

There are key pathophysiologic differences between UA/NSTEMI and STEMI that determine the specific treatment strategies for each type of ACS. As described in detail previously (see pages 14–25), UA/NSTEMI is a dynamic setting in which an unstable plaque “destabilizes” with erosion or rupture of the fibrous cap. This leads to exposure of tissue factor promoting adhesion and aggregation of platelets to form a platelet-rich plug. This platelet plug produces subtotal vessel occlusion causing resting ischaemia, the hallmark of UA. Often there is embolization of the platelet plug into the distal microcirculation producing small patches of myocardial necrosis and release of biomarkers, the NSTEMI. Similar to UA/NSTEMI, a STEMI is usually derived from an unstable plaque with platelet adhesion and aggregation. In contrast however, in STEMI the platelet core is stabilized by a mesh of cross-linked fibrin strands and trapped red blood cells producing total thrombotic occlusion of the infarct artery. The intracoronary thrombus associated with STEMI leads to a larger area of infarction and the need for alternate therapeutic strategies mandating rapid vessel reperfusion (Figure 46).

Risk stratification

Early risk stratification may help direct therapy for selected patients. When possible, patients at high risk should be directed/transported to a tertiary care hospital for possible revascularization and haemodynamic stabilization. Factors associated with high risk include advanced age, hypotension, tachycardia, heart failure and anterior wall MI. The TIMI group developed a useful simplified tool for estimating

Fig. 46 Diagnosis of STEMI.

The standard definitions of STEMI are:
1. Symptoms of myocardial ischaemia
2. ECG findings: > or =0.1 mV ST elevation in 2 or more contiguous ECG leads or new or presumed new left branch bundle block. Also true posterior MI may present with ST depression in V1, V2. A posterior MI quickly can be corroborated with bedside 2D transthoracic echo

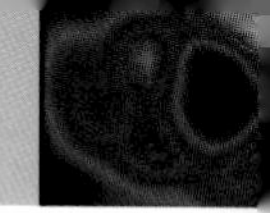

Risk index = (Heart rate x [Age/10]²)/Systolic blood pressure (mortality based on score with and without reperfusion)		
Risk Index	In-hospital mortality	30-day mortality
<12.5	0.6%	0.8%
>12.5–17.5	1.5%	1.9%
>17.5–22.5	3.1%	3.3%
>22.5–30	6.5%	7.3%
>30	15.8%	17.4%

Fig. 47 TIMI risk score for patients with STEMI. Adapted from Morrow DA, Antman EM, Giugliano RP, et al. A simple risk index for rapid initial triage of patients with ST-elevation myocardial infarction: an InTIME II substudy. Lancet 2001;358:1571–1575.

risk and adjusting treatment plans for patients with STEMI using age and vital signs (Figure 47).[156]

Prehospital assessment and treatment of chest pain (Figure 48)

Aspirin

As soon as MI is suspected aspirin should be ingested by the patient. The current recommendation is to chew and swallow nonenteric-coated aspirin 162–325 mg (in Europe the recommended doses are aspirin 150–325 mg).

Prehospital fibrinolysis

It has been recognized that from the onset of symptoms of acute coronary thrombosis there is a "golden hour" for reperfusion of myocardium at risk during which time there can be maximum salvage of myocardium.[157] This "time is muscle" concept has led to consideration of a strategy of prehospital fibrinolysis when feasible and safe. A meta-analysis of over 6000 patients randomized to prehospital versus traditional hospital initiated thrombolysis demonstrated that prehospital treatment shortens time to initiation of fibrinolysis by approximately 1 hour and reduces relative risk of all-cause mortality by 17%.[158] The ER-TIMI 19 study substantiated that prehospital fibrinolysis is feasible and can be safe with decreased time to reperfusion.[159] Alternatively immediate transfer to a facility for primary PCI should be considered when this option is available in a timely fashion. It should be emphasized that time to reperfusion is critical to improve patient outcomes, thus the treatment approach should be tailored to the strategy with the greatest likelihood of rapid reperfusion. Since reperfusion rates from fibrinolysis are highest when administered within 3 hours of onset of STEMI,[160] prehospital "lysis" may be preferred over transport for PCI. The CAPTIM study assessed the benefits of prehospital fibrinolysis versus transfer to a nearby facility for PCI. In this study primary angioplasty was not superior to pre-

"Prehospital fibrinolysis may accelerate reperfusion"

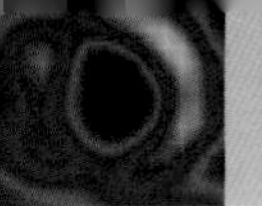

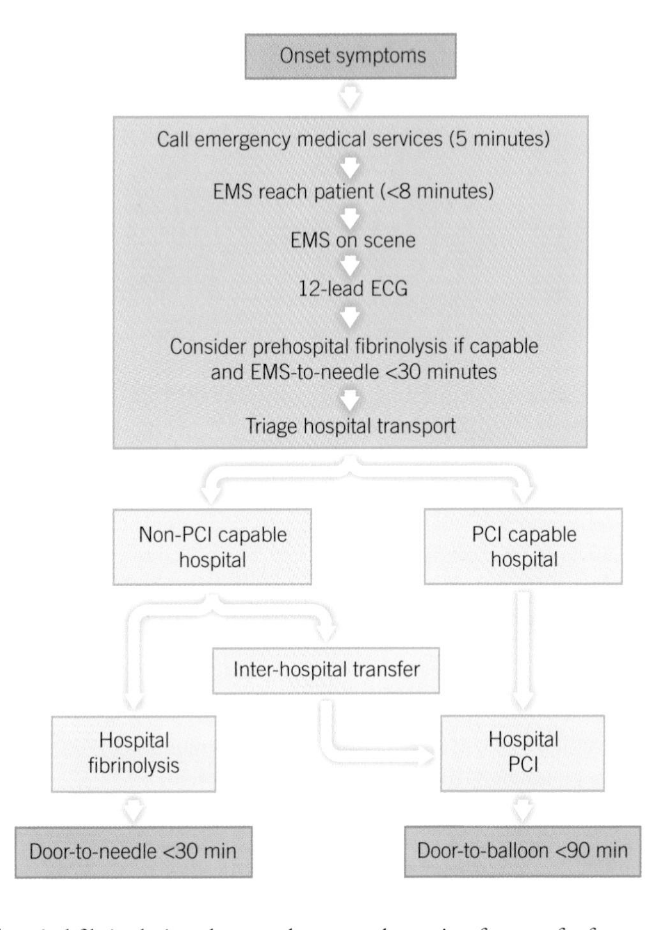

Fig. 48 Optimal prehospital treatment goals. Adapted from ACC/AHA Guidelines.[155]

hospital fibrinolysis as long as there was the option for transfer for possible rescue PCI.[161] The application of a prehospitalization fibrinolysis strategy requires a well-trained emergency medical services (EMS) team with off-site communication with hospital physicians. The ACC/AHA 2004 guidelines for the treatment of STEMI stress that the goal should be to keep ischaemic time within 120 minutes. For prehospital fibrinolysis they recommend a 30-minute maximum EMS-to-needle time. This should be followed by non-invasive assessment (symptoms and ECG) to determine if there is a need for rescue PCI.

“Choose a treatment strategy that keeps ischaemic time below 120 minutes”

Similar treatment goals have been set out in the UK Government's National Service Framework (NSF) for CHD, one objective being that 75% of eligible patients should receive fibrinolysis within 30 minutes of arrival at hospital. This has now been audited by the Myocardial Infarction National Audit Project (MINAP)[162] and shows that 89% of hospitals in England have achieved the within-30-minute goal in

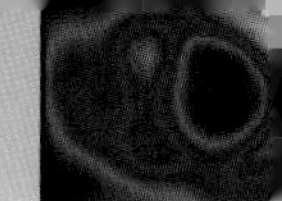

delivering lysis, which is a remarkable achievement for the UK National Health Service.

Medical therapy

Nitrates

Sublingual glyceryl trinitrate (nitroglycerin) 0.4 mg can be administered for ongoing chest pain. If pain persists after the initial dose a maximum of three doses can be administered over 20 minutes. Glyceryl trinitrate is contraindicated if the systolic blood pressure is less than 90 mmHg, heart rate is below 50 beats/minute or above 100 beats/minute, or there is suspected right ventricular infarction.

Intravenous glyceryl trinitrate has marginal benefits for treatment of STEMI. It may be helpful for patients who do not receive either PCI or fibrinolysis. Glyceryl trinitrate may also be beneficial for patients receiving fibrinolytics who have continued chest pain, persistent hypertension and/or left ventricular failure. The goal for iv glyceryl trinitrate is to titrate infusion rate to lower systolic pressure by 10% for normotensives and by 30% for hypertensives. Infusion is usually discontinued after 24–48 hours.

Oxygen

All patients should receive nasal oxygen at 2 litres/minute immediately and this should be continued until they are stabilized.

Analgesics

Morphine sulphate is the preferred analgesic agent to treat ongoing chest pain. The ACC/AHA guidelines recommend 2–4 mg iv with 2–8 mg increments every 5 to 15 minutes. European guidelines have similar recommendations of 4 to 8 mg morphine with additional doses of 2 mg at 5-minute intervals.

> *“Dual antiplatelet treatment with aspirin and clopidogrel for STEMI enhances coronary patency and reduces vessel reocclusion”*

Antiplatelet agents

As discussed above for prehospital treatment, patients should have immediate administration of non-enteric aspirin (162 mg or greater). Chewing and swallowing the aspirin enhances drug absorption. Clopidogrel can be considered as an alternative antiplatelet agent for aspirin-sensitive patients. Standard dosing is 75 mg/day. Clopidogrel however is a pro-drug, with a prolonged time to onset of action, thus a 300 mg loading dose is usually recommended to derive clinical benefit during the first few hours of treatment.[163] Patients likely to undergo PCI with stenting should receive a 300 mg loading dose of clopidogrel prior to or during cardiac catheterization. A 600 mg loading dose of clopidogrel may be superior to 300 mg but this has not been systematically tested in STEMI patients. Recent findings indicate that clopidogrel enhances reperfusion with thrombolytics.[163] Thus, it would be desirable to utilize a regimen that provides the most rapid antiplatelet effect that may augment reperfusion with PCI. Since many patients are resistant to individual antiplatelet medications, combined aspirin and clopidogrel may improve the chances of effective antiplatelet treatment. Dual antiplatelet therapy with aspirin plus clopidogrel has been shown to be a successful combination for NSTEMI in the CURE study. STEMI patients were studied in the recent CLARITY-TIMI 28 study which demonstrated improved coronary arterial patency when both antiplatelet drugs were added to fibrinolytic therapy and heparin.[164] Dual antiplatelet therapy (aspirin plus clopidogrel loading dose 300 mg followed by 75 mg/day) reduced the composite endpoint of coronary artery occlusion, death or recurrent MI from 21.7% to 15.0% (risk reduction [RR] 36%, 95% CI 24–47%, $p<0.001$). Prevention of coronary artery reocclusion was the most effected endpoint. The benefits of this combination of medications were not offset by excess major bleeding complications. This study however excluded patients over 75 years old or those with previous CABG. It is not known if addition of clopidogrel to aspirin improves clinical outcome in STEMI patients who receive an early invasive strategy since catheterization was delayed a median of 3.5 days in CLARITY. As with NSTEMI patients, the decision to administer clopidogrel should be delayed if emergency coronary bypass surgery is deemed a possibility.

“Oral beta-blockers are beneficial for most STEMI patients, though it may be preferable to delay initiation until the patient is haemodynamically stable”

Infarct size limitation

This section looks at evidence-based concomitant therapy for STEMI during the acute phase of hospital admission.

Beta-blockers

Intravenous beta-blockers are recommended as concomitant therapy with either fibrinolysis or PCI. Early use of beta-blockade reduces infarct size, incidence of reinfarction and ventricular arrhythmias. Most published experience has been with metoprolol. Initial iv dosing for metoprolol is 15 mg administered in 5 mg (slow 1–2 mg push) increments. If tolerated then immediately start oral metoprolol 25–50 mg every 12 hours. Alternatives to metoprolol are iv atenolol or esmolol. Esmolol is an ultra-short acting (half-life 7 minutes) beta-blocker that may be preferred for selected patients with mild left ventricular dysfunction. Dosing of esmolol is 50 μg/kg/minute with increments up to 200–300 μg/minute. Contraindications to beta-blockers in STEMI include:

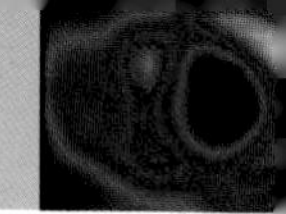

- bradycardia <60 beats/minute
- systolic blood pressure <100 mmHg
- moderate to severe heart failure or fluid overload
- heart block (any degree)
- bronchospasm or history of asthma.

Recent data from the COMMIT/CCS-2 trial cautions against the routine use of iv metoprolol in the first 24 hours of an acute MI.[165] In this 5-year joint China/UK trial of over 45,000 patients administration of three iv doses of 5 mg metoprolol followed by oral administration of metoprolol 200 mg daily resulted in an *increase* in the relative risk of cardiac shock by 30%, especially on the first day of treatment. While long-term use of oral beta-blockers after MI is beneficial, to minimize any potential hazard it may be best to delay initiation of beta-blockers for a few days, particularly for patients with Killip class II and III heart failure.

"Calcium antagonists have limited use in the acute phase of STEMI"

Calcium antagonists

Calcium antagonists do not provide added benefit to the treatment of STEMI. Nifedipine may actually worsen outcome. Intravenous diltiazem can be safely used to slow ventricular rate if the STEMI is complicated by rapid atrial fibrillation.

Renin-angiotensin-aldosterone inhibition

Patients with a large anterior MI or left ventricular failure should be considered for early treatment (within first 24 hours) with an oral ACE inhibitor. Both the GISSI-3 and ISIS-4 trials documented very early treatment benefit for a wide range of STEMI patients, especially those with Killip class >1.[166,167] The adverse effects of persistent hypotension and renal dysfunction are more common in ACE inhibitor treated patients, but the risks can be reduced by excluding patients with pre-existing hypotension (systolic pressure <100 mmHg or 30 mmHg or more below baseline) or significant renal failure. Initiation of therapy with a low dose of ACE inhibitor followed by gradual dose up-titration can minimize hypotension. Angiotensin receptor blockers (ARBs) can be considered as an alternative for renin-angiotensin blockade for patients with known side effects from an ACE inhibitor.

"Early administration of oral ACE inhibitors are beneficial in STEMI patients with anterior MI and/or heart failure"

Statins

Recent randomized clinical trials have provided solid evidence that intensive statin therapy is effective secondary prevention for patients presenting with ACS.[168–170] The mechanisms by which pre-hospital and in-hospital statin treatment may benefit ACS patients could be

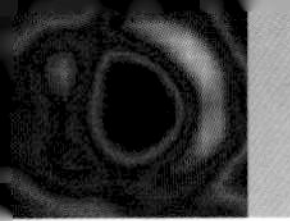

due to LDL lowering and/or the non-LDL (pleiotropic) effects of this class of medications.[171] The protective actions of statins may include: enhanced endothelial function (upregulation of e-NOS, lower VCAM and ICAM), anti-inflammatory effects (lower cytokines, IL-6, fibrinogen, CRP), lowered MMPs, and reduced tissue factor expression. The MIRACL trial randomized 3086 NSTEMI ACS patients to high-dose atorvastatin (80 mg/day) versus placebo.[168] At 4 months' follow-up the combined endpoint of death, non-fatal MI, cardiac arrest or recurrent ischaemia was reduced by 16% (RR 0.84, 95% CI 0.70–1.00, p=0.05). This benefit was primarily driven by lower recurrent ischaemia. MIRACL did not incorporate all current ACS therapies. Patients with PCI were excluded and there was low use of both GP IIb/IIIa inhibitors and clopidogrel. A more recent analysis of MIRACL[172] looked at whether plasma lipoproteins at baseline and then at 6 weeks after randomization, predicted outcome. This showed that high-density lipoprotein (HDL), but not LDL, cholesterol measured at the initial stage of the ACS predicts the risk of recurrent cardiovascular events in the ensuing 16 weeks (Figure 49). This suggests that the clinical benefit of atorvastatin after ACS might be mediated via non-lipid or pleiotropic effects of the statin.

Fig. 49 Relationship between time to first occurence of a primary clinical endpoint up to 16 weeks after randomization and baseline, Week 6, and Week 0 to Week 6 absolute change values. Reproduced from Olsson AG, Schwartz GG, Szarek M, et al. Eur Heart J 2005;26:890–896. By permission of Oxford University Press.

Lipid parameter	Hazard ratio	95% CI
LDL-C		
Baseline value	1.000	0.997, 1.003
Week 6 value	1.001	0.995, 1.006
Absolute change	1.001	0.995, 1.007
HDL-C		
Baseline value	0.986	0.979, 0.994
Week 6 value	0.988	0.973, 1.004
Absolute change	0.992	0.976, 1.008
Total cholesterol		
Baseline value	0.999	0.996, 1.001
Week 6 value	0.999	0.994, 1.003
Absolute change	1.001	0.996, 1.005
Triglycerides		
Baseline value	1.000	0.999, 1.001
Week 6 value	0.999	0.997, 1.001
Absolute change	1.001	0.999, 1.003
ApoB		
Baseline value	1.002	0.999, 1.005
ApoA–1		
Baseline value	0.993	0.990, 0.997

Hazard ratios with 95% confidence intervals

0.97 0.98 0.99 1.00 1.01 1.02 1.03

Hazard ratio for 1 mg/dL increase in lipid parameter

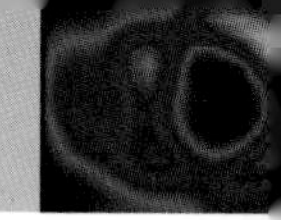

The PROVE IT trial compared two statin regimens in over 4000 ACS patients: moderate lipid lowering with pravastatin 40 mg/day versus intensive therapy using atorvastatin 80 mg/day.[169] Drugs were initiated around time of discharge. After 2 years' follow-up the intensive treatment arm had a lower incidence of the combined primary endpoint of death, non-fatal MI, UA, and stroke compared with the moderate statin treatment arm (reduced hazard ratio 16%, 95% CI 5–26%, p=0.005). In contrast to MIRACL, 69% of PROVE IT patients had revascularization prior to randomization. The recent A to Z trial randomized nearly 4500 ACS patients to either early intensive statin treatment (simvastatin 40 mg/day for 30 days followed by 80 mg/day) or a delayed less intensive statin regimen (placebo for 4 months followed by simvastatin 20 mg).[170] Though there was no difference in the primary endpoint (cardiovascular death, non-fatal MI, stroke, readmission for ACS) at 4 months, improved outcome was noted in the early/intensive dose statin group in the 4- to 24-month follow-up period (hazard ratio 0.75, 95% CI 0.60–0.95, p=0.02). Concomitant therapy in A to Z was different from that used in MIRACL and PROVE IT. A to Z and PROVE IT had high use of GP IIb/IIIa inhibitors and in A to Z only 44% of patients had PCI prior to randomization.

These data strongly suggest that early intensive statin treatment should be routinely administered to the high-risk ACS patient. The optimal timing for initiation of statin therapy in the setting of ACS (e.g. immediate in-hospital versus at discharge) has not been determined. In an animal model of MI, pretreatment with a statin resulted in reduced ischaemic injury.[173] In man this therapy appears effective when started after stabilization with antiplatelet agents, GP IIb/IIIa inhibitors and revascularization. The MIRACL trial started administering statin therapy 24 to 96 hours (mean 63 hours) after admission. PROVE-IT randomized statins at a median of 7 days after onset of ACS. A to Z started statins after initial stabilization for at least 12 hours but no longer than 5 days (mean 3.7 days). GRACE suggests an advantage to very early administration (<48 hours) of statins in ACS patients.[174] GRACE observed that patients on statins both pre- and during hospitalization presented with less ST elevation and had fewer MIs. Furthermore, patients given statins in hospital, with or without prehospital statin use, had lower mortality compared with patients who never received statins prior to discharge (OR 0.66, 95% CI 0.56–0.77). In contrast, patients on statins prehospitalization who had statins discontinued upon admission had similar mortality to those who had no statins prior to or during hospitalization. Most importantly patients started on statins in hospital had lower mortality and fewer combined

“Early statin therapy, prior to hospital discharge, should be considered for all patients with STEMI”

adverse events (death, in-hospital MI, stroke) compared with patients who did not receive statins prior to discharge (OR 0.38, 95% CI 0.30–0.48 versus OR 0.87, 95% CI 0.78–0.97). These benefits were marginal however, after adjustment for hospital of admission (RR 0.81, 95% CI 0.65–1.1).

Clinical trials have established that intensive high-dose statin therapy is beneficial post ACS (MIRACL and PROVE IT). While very early use of statins in hospital for ACS patients has not undergone evidence-based study, the safety appears sound. Even though precise timing of initiation of statins remains unanswered, it is clear that intensive statin therapy should be the standard of care prior to or at discharge.

Reperfusion options for treatment of STEMI: general issues

General principles of reperfusion therapy

"The goal for door-to-needle or door-to-medical contact time is <30 minutes for initiation of a fibrinolytic drug"

Rapid reperfusion of the occluded infarct vessel with either fibrinolysis or PCI is the major goal of treatment that results in improved patient outcome. It is critical to select the reperfusion strategy that will minimize time to reperfusion by keeping the medical contact-to-needle or contact–to-balloon time as short as possible. Reperfusion options include:

1. Thrombolytic monotherapy.
2. Thrombolysis plus GP IIb/IIIa inhibition.
3. Primary PCI.
4. Facilitated PCI (reduced dose thrombolytic plus a GP IIb/IIIa inhibitor prior to PCI).

Urgent reperfusion therapy should be given in the case of ST-elevation new Q waves or new or presumed new left bundle branch block. Reperfusion therapy, if clinically warranted, should not be delayed for enzyme results to be obtained.

Early reperfusion reduces myocardial infarct size and improves survival but preservation of myocardium and mortality reduction are dependent on both rapid and full restoration of epicardial coronary artery flow. The TIMI flow grade achieved with thrombolytics (TIMI flow grade 0=no flow, 1=slight flow, 2=moderate flow, and 3=brisk flow) correlates with mortality. A meta-analysis published by Anderson *et al* reported 30-day mortality of 8.8% with TIMI grade 0/1, 7.0% with TIMI grade 2, and 3.7% with TIMI grade 3.[175]

Improved epicardial blood flow with TIMI grade 3 pattern alone does not predict improved outcome. Despite successful reperfusion of the epicardial coronary there can be poor tissue perfusion of the myocardium in the zone at risk for infarction. Up to 25% of STEMI

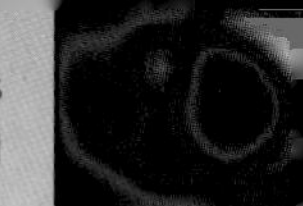

patients treated with early PCI have impaired coronary microcirculation due to the "no-reflow" phenomenon. The mechanisms of "no-reflow" are only partially understood and may be due to either:
1. Reperfusion injury.
2. Microvascular obstruction.

Reperfusion injury appears to be a complex interaction of leukocytes, platelets and endothelial cells that cause pro-oxidant stress and myocyte injury. Plaque rupture activates platelets that cause enhanced expression of neutrophil adhesion molecules. This leads to leukocyte infiltration of the adjacent myocardial cells where the activated leukocytes release oxygen free radicals thereby causing tissue damage. Microvascular obstruction occurs from:
1. Distal embolization of platelet-rich thrombi into the capillary bed.
2. Progressive leukocyte entrapment in capillaries.
3. Spasm of distal arterioles.

"No-reflow" is a predictor of poor outcome with increased morbidity and mortality after either thrombolysis or PCI.[110,176] Lowest mortality is seen when there is both angiographic TIMI 3 flow (epicardial) plus rapid dye clearing from the at-risk myocardial (microvascular) zone. Microvascular obstruction can be semiquantified at catheterization as persistent or delayed dye clearance in the myocardium distal to the reperfused vascular segment. Using both angiographic criteria mortality was reported as 0.7% for patients with both TIMI 3 flow and brisk myocardial perfusion pattern versus 10.9% mortality for patients with only TIMI 3 flow but no brisk myocardial perfusion pattern ($p<0.001$).[110]

It is critical to restore TIMI 3 flow as early as possible since mortality increases with each 15 minute delay.[177,178] To maximize outcome the recommended door-to-needle or medical contact-to-needle time for administration of a fibrinolytic medication is <30 minutes. For reperfusion with PCI both the AHA and the ESC have set the goal for medical contact-to-balloon or door-to-balloon time as 90 minutes. Fibrinolysis should be administered if PCI is not available; or delay until PCI is expected since there is a strong correlation between symptom onset-to-balloon time and outcome.

"To maximize outcome the recommended door-to-needle or medical contact-to-needle time for administration of a fibrinolytic medication is <30 minutes"

Patient selection for thrombolytic monotherapy

Patient selection for fibrinolysis is mainly determined by the time elapsed from the onset of symptoms to presentation for medical treatment. Optimal benefit from thrombolytic therapy is gained when drug is administered within 12 hours of onset symptoms. The concept of the first "golden hour", whereby a significant reduction in mortality can be achieved with very early treatment, was investigated by

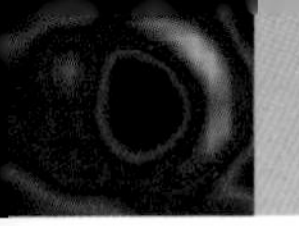

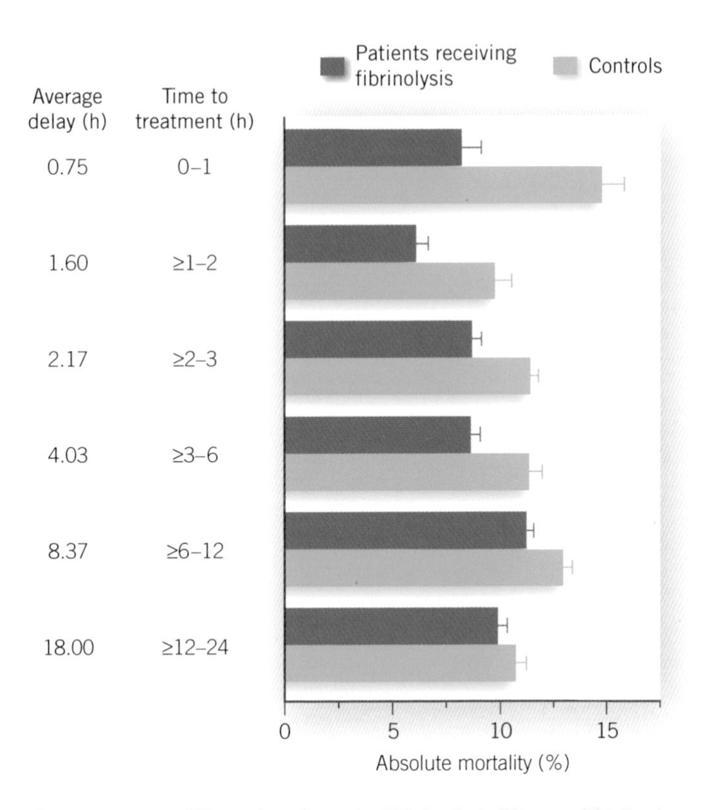

Fig. 50 Mortality at 35 days among fibrinolytic-treated and control patients, according to treatment delay. Adapted from Boersma E, Maas ACP, Deckers JW, Simoons ML. Early thrombolytic treatment in acute myocardial infarction: reappraisal of the golden hour. Lancet 1996;348:771–775. © Elsevier

“Thrombolytics can be beneficial for patients within 12 hours from the onset of symptoms”

Boersma *et al.*[179] Using data from the Fibrinolytic Therapy Trialists' Collaborative Group study of over 50,000 patients in randomized trials that compared fibrinolytic therapy with placebo or control they were able to show the absolute reduction in mortality was greatest among patients who presented within 1 hour of symptom onset (Figure 50) with 65 lives saved per 1000 patients treated at 35 days. Benefit was also higher in patients randomized in the second hour, with 37 lives saved per 1000 patients treated. The benefit per 1000 treated in subgroups presenting at ≥2–3 hours, ≥3–6 hours, ≥6–12 hours, and ≥12–24 hours, was 26, 29, 18, and 9, respectively.

Partial benefit may be obtained when fibrinolytics are given 12–24 hours post onset of symptoms but only if there is persistent chest pain and ST elevation >0.1 mV in two or more contiguous precordial leads or two limb leads (ACC/AHA 2004 Guidelines).[58]

Contraindications for fibrinolytics

Absolute and relative contraindications to thrombolytic therapy are listed in Figure 51. Patients with significant (≥4%) risk of intracranial haemorrhage should undergo PCI rather than thrombolytic therapy.

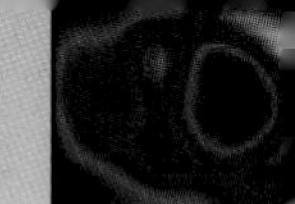

Absolute contraindications to thrombolysis:
1. Any prior intracranial haemorrhage
2. Known structural cerebrovascular lesion or neoplasm
3. Ischaemic stroke within 3 months except if within 3 hours
4. Suspected aortic dissection
5. Active bleeding or bleeding diathesis (not including menses)
6. Closed head or facial trauma in past 3 months
Relative contraindications for thrombolytic drugs:
1. Chronic severe, poorly controlled hypertension
2. Severe hypertension at presentation (systolic blood pressure >180 mmHg or diastolic blood pressure >110 mmHg)
3. History of ischaemic stroke greater than 3 months, dementia, other intracranial pathology
4. Traumatic or prolonged (<10 minutes) cardiopulmonary arrest
5. Major surgery within past 3 weeks
6. Recent internal bleeding (2–4 weeks)
7. Non-compressible vascular puncture
8. Pregnancy
9. Active peptic ulcer
10. Current use of anticoagulants
11. Prior allergy or exposure (>5 days) to streptokinase if using streptokinase again

Fig. 51 Relative and absolute contraindications to thrombolysis. Reproduced with permission from Antman EM, Anbe DT, Armstrong PW, et al. ACC/AHA guidelines for the management of patients with ST-elevation myocardial infarction: A report of the American College of Cardiology/American Heart Association Task Force on Practice Guidelines (Committee to Revise the 1999 Guidelines for the Management of patients with acute myocardial infarction). J Am Coll Cardiol 2004;44:E1–E211. © Elsevier

Fibrinolytic therapy versus primary PCI

Whereas fibrinolytic therapy has the advantage of immediate and easy administration, primary PCI provides higher rates of reperfusion with a lower risk of reinfarction and major bleeding, especially intracranial haemorrhage. Meta-analysis of 23 trials comparing early primary PCI with early fibrinolysis demonstrated a significant advantage of PCI for short-term (4–6 weeks) endpoints including overall mortality, non-fatal reinfarction, stroke, and the combined triple endpoint.[180] PCI provides the greatest mortality reduction versus fibrinolysis in patients with cardiogenic shock and heart failure. Fibrinolytics are particularly effective when administered early, especially within 2 hours of chest pain onset. Over time, however, thrombus resistance to fibrinolysis develops and the ability to achieve TIMI 3 reperfusion with thrombolytics diminishes significantly. Patients presenting beyond 2 hours have superior outcome with PCI. Overall, primary PCI achieves early TIMI 3 flow in 70–90% of patients; whereas early fibrinolysis only achieves TIMI 2/3 flow in 50–60% of patients. In addition early reocclusion rate after PCI is very low, in the range of 5% after

“PCI is preferred over thrombolysis for patients within 12 hours from the onset of symptoms if medical contact-to-balloon or door-to-balloon time can be achieved in <90 minutes”

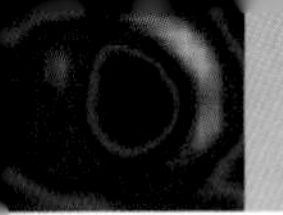

stenting.[181] The benefit of PCI, however, is highly dependent on a readily available catheterization team with a short door-to-balloon time. The GUSTO-IIb trial showed that 30-day mortality was lowest in patients treated with PCI within 60 minutes and was progressively higher in those who experienced incremental treatment delays.[182] Based on this evidence both the ESC[57] and the ACC/AHA[58] recommend PCI for patients presenting within 12 hours of chest pain onset when catheterization and balloon inflation can be performed within 90 minutes from first medical contact. This approach is preferred even if transfer to a tertiary care centre is required.

Though the optimal time window of benefit from PCI is within 12 hours of onset of symptoms, PCI may be offered to patients 12–24 hours post onset of symptoms who have any of:

- severe heart failure
- haemodynamic or electrical instability
- continuing symptoms of ischaemia.

Late PCI >12 hours after onset of chest pain has been shown to have small, but real, benefit for symptomatic patients.[183]

“PCI may be beneficial 12–24 hours after onset of symptoms in patients with ongoing ischaemia or electrical or haemodynamic instability”

Patient selection for primary PCI

The specific patient categories recommended to receive PCI in the 2004 updated ACC/AHA Guidelines for STEMI are shown in Figure 52. Primary PCI is not recommended for stable, asymptomatic patients >12 hours from onset of MI. In clinically stable patients, only the infarct artery should be stented during the initial catheterization.

Primary PCI without on-site cardiac surgery may be considered at a hospital that has an experienced interventional cardiology team that has a backup option for rapid transfer to a nearby hospital with cardiac surgery capability.

Fig. 52 Specific patient categories recommended to receive PCI in the 2004 updated ACC/AHA Guidelines for STEMI. Based upon ACC/AHA 2004 Guidelines.[58]

1. Symptoms <3 hours duration with expected door-to-balloon time (PCI reperfusion) 1 hour or less long than door-to-needle time (administration of thrombolytic).
2. Symptoms >3 hours and medical contact-to-balloon or door-to-balloon time <90 minutes.
3. Patients <75 years old who are <36 hours from onset of MI and within <18 hours' duration of shock. PCI should also be considered for selected patients >75 years old.
4. Patients with severe heart failure who have ongoing MI <12 hours and can be reperfused in <90 minutes of contact.
5. Ongoing symptoms 12–24 hours with either severe CHF, haemodynamic instability, or continuing ischaemic symptoms.

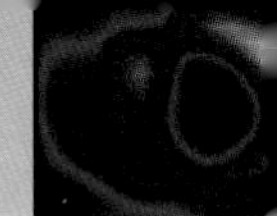

Facilitated PCI

Patients with STEMI admitted to community hospitals *without* PCI capability have several treatment options:

- fibrinolysis alone
- immediate transfer to a tertiary care hospital for PCI
- facilitated PCI.

Facilitated PCI comprises initial medical treatment with fibrinolytics (usually at a reduced dose) and/or GP IIb/IIIa inhibitor to achieve early partial infarct vessel reperfusion followed by immediate transfer to an institution for early PCI to ensure TIMI grade 3 flow reperfusion. This combined approach may maximize myocardial salvage and minimize mortality especially when there is transport delay for PCI. It has been shown that a small amount of flow in the infarct-related vessel prior to intervention has enhanced outcome in STEMI patients treated with PCI.[184] Early administration of a GP IIb/IIIa inhibitor alone may produce TIMI flow grade 3 reperfusion in 30% of patients.[185,186] The potential downside of initial thrombolytic plus GP IIb/IIIa followed by PCI is the risk of major bleeding. Bleeding risk may be mitigated by administration of half dose thrombolytic but more safety data are needed to analyse this risk. Unanswered is whether or not facilitation will benefit patients presenting 2 to 3 hours after onset of symptoms. Pilot trials of facilitated PCI are encouraging for this approach, however definitive trials await publication.[187]

Reperfusion: fibrinolytic agents

The ideal fibrinolytic is an agent that produces rapid, complete reperfusion with a low rate of reocclusion. Administration should be simple with low risk of severe bleeding and antigenicity. Follow-up PCI or CABG surgery should be possible and the cost of the agent should be low. Clinical assessment of the efficacy of fibrinolytics in achieving high grade reperfusion can be estimated by serial assessment of chest pain and ECGs for tracking evolution of ST elevation.

“Streptokinase should be limited to STEMI patients with symptoms of less than 12 hours’ duration”

Selection of fibrinolytics

Fibrinolytics are classified as non-fibrin specific (streptokinase, anistreplase, urokinase) or fibrin specific (alteplase, reteplase, tenecteplase).

Streptokinase was the first thrombolytic agent shown to benefit ACS patients with either STEMI or new bundle branch block. Clinical studies have shown time-dependent improvement of outcome using streptokinase. Treatment <6 hours from onset of symptoms can save 30 lives per 1000 patients treated; whereas treatment with streptokinase at 7 to 12 hours post onset of chest pain can save 20 lives per 1000 patients treated. Late treatment using streptokinase 13–18 hours

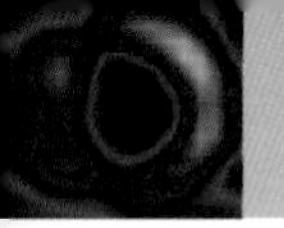

Fig. 53 Comparison of fibrin-specific fibrinolytic agents.

	Alteplase	Reteplase	Tenecteplase
Half-life	<5 minutes	13–16 minutes	20–24 minutes
Administration	Infusion	Double bolus	Single bolus
Weight adjusted	Yes	No	Yes
Fibrin affinity	+++	30% of alteplase	14x alteplase
Clot penetration	+	++	+

post onset of chest pain may save 10 lives per 1000 patients treated but this gain is offset by four strokes with high mortality or morbidity resulting in a recommendation to limit streptokinase to patients with onset of symptoms within 12 hours.[188] A recent study[189] conducted in Germany highlighted wide variations in the activity, purity, and composition among the 16 preparations of streptokinase from 11 manufacturers that were tested. Such findings have potentially serious clinical implications.

“Fibrin-specific fibrinolytic agents are preferred over streptokinase for STEMI patients treated >4 hours after onset of symptoms”

Alteplase was the first of the second generation fibrinolytics that have the added pharmacologic property of fibrin affinity. Alteplase was compared with streptokinase in the GUSTO-I study.[190] Patients treated with alteplase had lower mortality than the streptokinase-treated group (absolute RR 1.1%, relative RR 14%). The small benefit of alteplase over streptokinase was attributed to a higher frequency of early (90 minute) patency obtained with alteplase. TIMI grade 3 flow was achieved in only 32% of streptokinase-treated patients compared with 54% receiving alteplase.[191]

Two mutant fibrin-specific agents have been developed with longer half-lives than alteplase. Reteplase has a prolonged half-life permitting double-bolus administration rather than the continuous infusion required with alteplase. Clot adhesion and penetration exceeds that of alteplase resulting in potentially greater coronary patency. Reteplase has been compared with alteplase for reperfusion and mortality. In RAPID-I TIMI grade 3 flow rate was 62.7% with reteplase compared with 49.3% with alteplase.[192] The GUSTO III trial evaluated clinical outcome of STEMI patients randomized to either reteplase or alteplase and 30-day mortality was equal between the two treatments.[193]

Tenecteplase is the most recently developed fibrinolytic agent and has the advantage of an even longer half-life allowing administration as a single bolus. This makes it feasible to administer as prehospital thrombolysis, perhaps by ambulance crews and other suitably trained

Drug	Dosing	Features
Streptokinase	1.5 million units over 30–60 minutes	Lower reperfusion rate than fibrin-specific agents, lowest cost
Alteplase	15 mg bolus – then 0.75 mg/kg over 30 minutes (maximum 50 mg) – then 0.50 mg/kg over 60 minutes (maximum 35 mg)	Lower mortality than streptokinase Short half-life requires infusion adjustment
Tenecteplase	Weight-based single bolus over 10 seconds <60 kg = 30 mg 60–69 kg = 35 mg 70–79 kg = 40 mg 80–89 kg = 45 mg >90 kg = 50 mg	Efficacy similar to alteplase with lower bleeding complications when weight adjusted
Reteplase	10 units over 2 minutes – then repeat 10 units at 30 minutes	Efficacy similar to alteplase

Fig. 54 Fibrinolytic drug administration. These fibrinolytic regimens for acute MI are the same in US and European guidelines, and aspirin should be given to all patients without contraindications.

paramedics. It also has an improved safety and efficacy profile due to increased fibrin specificity permitting less systemic fibrinolysis with less bleeding and greater clot lysis potential.[194] Dosing needs to be weight-based to minimize bleeding complications. The TIMI 10B study compared tenecteplase with accelerated alteplase and found 90-minute TIMI flow grade 3 patency to be equal for the two medications.[195] Rate of bleeding was lower with tenecteplase versus alteplase in TIMI 10B. The ASSENT-2 trial compared mortality with tenecteplase versus alteplase.[196] Survival was similar with both fibrinolytic medications. Rates of haemorrhagic stroke and other major bleeding were similar between both groups. ASSENT-3[197] looked at the safety of full-dose tenecteplase in combination with enoxaparin, abciximab, or weight-adjusted UFH. There were significantly fewer efficacy endpoints (including death, reinfarction, refractory ischaemia, intracranial haemorrhage or major bleeding) in the enoxaparin and abciximab groups than in the UFH group. The combination of enoxaparin and tenecteplase emerged as "the best treatment in this trial" and warrants further study as an alternative reperfusion strategy in the future. Patient enrolment into ASSENT 4, a randomized exploratory Phase IIIb/IV clinical study of single-bolus tenecteplase in combination with an early planned PCI versus PCI alone in patients with acute MI, was suspended following a planned interim data review (May 2005). This

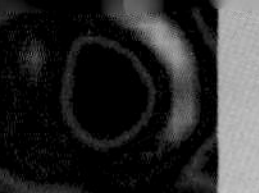

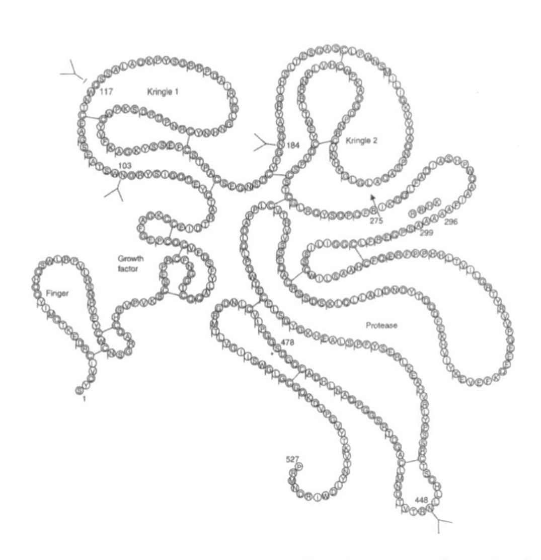

Fig. 55 The structure of tenecteplase. Tenecteplase has been called the TNK-mutant of alteplase. It consists of the alteplase molecule with the exception of three point mutations at positions 103, 117, and 296–299. Picture courtesy of Boehringer-Ingelheim.

showed higher mortality in those treated with tenecteplase plus heparin followed by PCI than in the heparin plus PCI-alone arm. The higher mortality was consistent with that seen in large-scale thrombolysis trials and not due to excess bleeding or higher rates of intracranial haemorrhage, which were comparable to previous fibrinolytic trials.

“The three fibrin-specific thrombolytic agents have similar efficacy and safety, however tenecteplase was superior to alteplase in patients treated >4 hours after onset of symptoms in one large clinical trial”

Fibrinolytic drugs comparison summary

The non-fibrin specific fibrinolytic streptokinase is an inexpensive medication with slightly lower reperfusion rates and mortality compared with the fibrin-specific agents. Fibrin-specific agents are expensive but they appear to have enhanced efficacy over streptokinase for STEMI patients treated >4 hours after onset of symptoms.[198] The three fibrin-specific fibrinolytic agents have equal clinical efficacy and safety profiles, though tenecteplase has shown improved outcome compared with alteplase in patients treated >4 hours.[196] The fibrinolytic medications that can be administered by bolus have the advantages of ease of use, shorter door-to-drug time, potential for pre-hospital treatment, and fewer medication errors.

Adjunctive therapies

Antiplatelet therapy

Fibrinolytic therapy for the management of acute STEMI is limited by inadequate reperfusion or thrombotic reocclusion in approximately 25% of patients and the presence of an occluded artery after fibrinolysis is associated with a doubling of long-term mortality. The benefit of additional antiplatelet therapy with clopidogrel in the acute management of STEMI has recently been demonstrated in two large

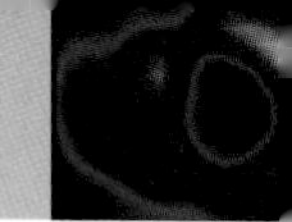

clinical trials. The CLARITY-TIMI 28 trial,[164] demonstrated that the use of clopidogrel (300 mg loading dose followed by 75 mg/day) resulted in a 36% reduction in the composite endpoint of an occluded artery, death or recurrent MI prior to angiography (average 3.5 days) or at hospital discharge if angiography was not performed (average 8 days). At 30 days the use of clopidogrel among patients who received fibrinolytic therapy reduced the incidence of cardiovascular death, recurrent MI or recurrent ischaemia leading to urgent revascularization by 20%. The use of clopidogrel reduced the need for urgent angiography <48 hours of STEMI by 21% and the need for GP IIb/IIIa use if PCI was performed by 16%. The beneficial effects of clopidogrel were observed irrespective of whether a fibrin-specific lytic was used or whether UFH or LMWH was used as an adjunctive anticoagulant.

“Consider dual antiplatelet therapy (aspirin + clopidogrel) for STEMI patients when there is a delay to PCI”

The findings in CLARITY were supported by the much larger COMMIT/CCS2 trial[165] which evaluated the use of clopidogrel 75 mg daily (without a high loading dose) on clinical outcomes at hospital discharge (on average 16 days). The use of clopidogrel was associated with a significant 7% relative risk reduction in death from all causes and a 9% risk reduction in death, recurrent MI or stroke. These benefits were observed across a range of subgroups and importantly the benefit of even this low loading dose was observed irrespective of time from onset of initial symptoms. Taken together these two recent trials support the use of clopidogrel as adjunctive therapy to fibrinolysis in STEMI. This treatment may be particularly beneficial to sites who are not performing primary PCI.

“Clopidogrel 300 mg could be used as adjunctive therapy in patients receiving fibrinolytic therapy followed by a maintenance dose of 75 mg for at least 30 days in patients undergoing primary PCI for STEMI”

In patients receiving primary PCI for treatment of STEMI a loading dose of 300 mg of clopidogrel is the dose of choice in the US but in Europe a 600 mg dose is now preferred and recommended.[105] Although not in the current clinical guidelines the use of clopidogrel for 30 days as adjunctive therapy to pharmacological treatment in STEMI reduces cardiovascular risk.

Heparin therapy

The theoretic advantage of adding heparin to thrombolytic therapy is to enhance vessel patency and prevent coronary re-thrombosis. Additional benefits may include prevention of left ventricular thrombi, pulmonary emboli and deep venous thrombosis. However, evidence-based data for clinical benefit from adjunctive heparin in the setting of concomitant aspirin are lacking.

Unfractionated heparin

Patients treated with streptokinase are recommended to receive UFH especially if they are at high risk for emboli (anterior MI, prior emboli,

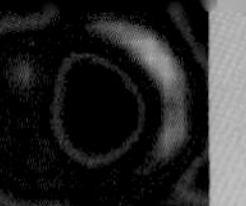

atrial fibrillation, or left ventricular thrombus). There is no consensus for use of UFH in patients treated with a fibrin-specific fibrinolytic agent. The 2004 *ACC/AHA Guidelines for the Management of Patients with STEMI*[155] do not recommend routine use of UFH with these second generation thrombolytics. In contrast the *7th ACCP Conference on Antithrombotic and Thrombolytic Therapy: Evidence-based Guidelines* recommend weight-adjusted UFH for 48 hours (level of evidence Grade 1C).[199]

Recommended dosing of UFH is summarized below:

- *Heparin infusion protocol for patients receiving streptokinase:* All patients should receive an initial iv bolus of UFH 5000 units. This is followed by an infusion of 1000 units/hour for patients >80 kg, or 800 units/hour for patients <80 kg. Target aPTT is 50–75 seconds. Alternatively subcutaneous heparin can be administered 12,500 units/12 hours. In patients who have HIT bivalirudin may be considered as an alternative agent.
- *Heparin infusion protocol with fibrin-specific agents:* The dosing protocol for UFH should be weight adjusted: bolus 60 units/kg (maximum 4000 units). Follow-up infusion 12 units/kg/hour (maximum 1000 units/kg/hour); target aPTT 50–75 seconds.

“STEMI patients may not need heparin when treatment includes a fibrinolytic plus aspirin”

Low molecular weight heparin

Enoxaparin and dalteparin have shown promise as alternatives to UFH in small to intermediate size trials. The largest study to date has been the ASSENT-3 trial, which compared full-dose tenecteplase plus either enoxaparin or weight-adjusted UFH.[197] No difference was observed for rates of intracranial haemorrhage, severe bleeding or 30-day mortality between the LMWH and the UFH treated groups. Larger randomized trials are needed to determine a specific recommendation for LMWH in STEMI patients.

GP IIb/IIIa inhibitors

A limitation of fibrinolytic drugs is that the ability to lyse fibrin from the fibrin-thrombin clot exposes free thrombin that paradoxically stimulates platelet aggregation leading to possible drug resistance, arterial reocclusion and microembolization of the downstream microcirculation. Therefore the combination of a fibrinolytic plus a GP IIb/IIIa inhibitor should theoretically enhance TIMI flow and TIMI myocardial perfusion grades over fibrinolytic monotherapy. GP IIb/IIIa inhibitors allow for a reduced dose of fibrinolytic and may facilitate subsequent PCI. The GUSTO V study compared half-dose reteplase plus abciximab to full-dose reteplase.[200] Combination therapy reduced non-fatal

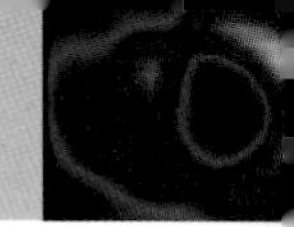

reinfarction and complications of MI but there was no difference in total mortality. Though intracranial haemorrhage rates were similar, combination therapy led to increased moderate-to-severe bleeding predominantly in patients >75 years. Similar results were observed in the ASSENT-3 trial with half-dose tenecteplase plus abciximab.[197]

A meta-analysis showed that abciximab was associated with a significant reduction in short- and long-term mortality when utilized as part of a primary angioplasty strategy, but not in conjunction with fibrinolysis.[201] While the largest body of clinical outcomes data is available for abciximab in the STEMI setting, patency rates and rates of TIMI grade 3 flow for eptifibatide and tirofiban are similar to those of abciximab.[202,203] A higher dose of tirofiban was evaluated in the STRATEGY trial of STEMI patients undergoing primary PCI and no difference in death or recurrent MI was observed between abciximab and tirofiban.[126] We recommend that patients transferred for primary PCI receive a heparinoid (UFH or LMWH) and an iv GP IIb/IIIa inhibitor prior to transfer. The bulk of evidence does not presently support use of combination fibrinolytic and GP IIb/IIIa inhibition prior to primary PCI given the higher risk of bleeding and intracranial haemorrhage, particularly among those over age 75 years.[204]

The latest ACC/AHA guidelines give a class IIb indication to the combination of a GP IIa/IIIb inhibitor plus half-dose reteplase or tenecteplase to reduce reinfarction in patients <75 years old, anterior MI and low-bleeding risk.[155,205] This strategy may also be preferred when early PCI is planned. Pharmacological facilitation of PCI (half-dose thrombolytic plus a GP IIb/IIIa inhibitor followed by PCI) is discussed below.

> *"Risk factors for intracranial haemorrhage complicating thrombolysis include age, female gender, history of cerebrovascular accident, hypertension and low body weight"*

Complications of thrombolytic therapy

Intracranial haemorrhage

Intracranial haemorrhage occurs in 0.5% to 0.9% of patients receiving fibrinolytic monotherapy with up to 2/3 mortality. Patient selection and appropriate drug dosing can minimize this risk. Risk factors for intracranial haemorrhage include:[206,207]

- age >75 years (OR 4.34; 95% CI 3.45–5.45)
- female gender (OR 1.56; 95% CI 1.31–1.92)
- history of prior stroke (OR 1.90; 95% CI 1.37–2.65)
- diastolic blood pressure >100 mmHg (OR 1.40; 95% CI 1.12–1.99)
- systolic blood pressure >160 mmHg (OR 1.48; 95% CI 1.14–1.92)
- alteplase dose >1.5 mg/kg (OR 1.49; 95% CI 1.22–1.84)
- low body weight.

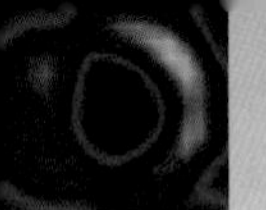

If the patient manifests any neurologic changes during treatment intracranial haemorrhage must be ruled out. Fibrinolytics, antiplatelet drugs and anticoagulants should be discontinued until obtaining brain imaging and further neurologic evaluation. It may be necessary to reverse the effects of haematologically active drugs with cryo-precipitate, fresh frozen plasma, protamine or platelet transfusions.

Elective PCI after fibrinolysis

Elective PCI is often performed hours, days or weeks after successful thrombolytic therapy. PCI of the residual infarct-related residual stenosis within the initial 48 hours following successful fibrinolysis is not usually beneficial unless there is recurrent ischaemia. Late PCI was compared with routine medical therapy in the DANAMI-2 trial.[208] In this study of 1572 STEMI patients with rest or stress-induced ischaemia, who were randomized to PCI or accelerated treatment with iv alteplase, PCI-treated patients had less UA and non-fatal MI (Figure 56).

Other high-risk groups that are candidates for PCI include patients with low ejection fraction (<0.40), heart failure (even with preserved ejection fractions), or life-threatening ventricular arrhythmias. Routine invasive strategy for *all* patients post successful fibrinolysis has a class IIb recommendation from the 2004 ACC/AHA guidelines.[155]

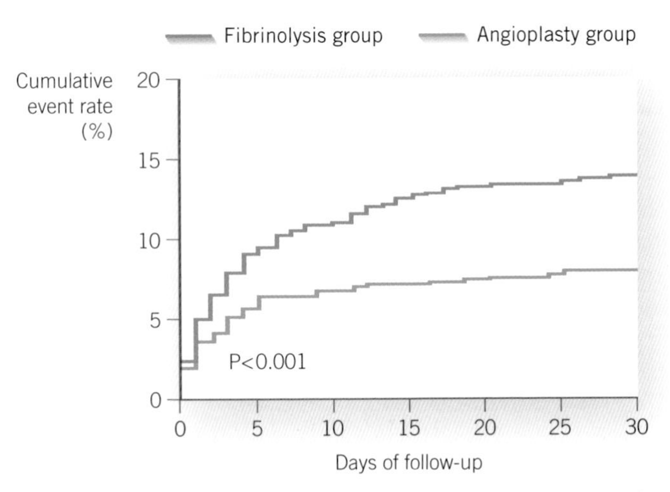

Fig. 56 Kaplan-Meier curves showing cumulative event rates for the primary composite endpoint of death, clinical reinfarction, or disabling stroke during 30 days of follow-up. Reproduced with permission from Andersen HR, Nielsen TT, Rasmussen K, et al. A comparison of coronary angioplasty with fibrinolytic therapy in acute myocardial infarction. N Engl J Med 2003;349:733–742.

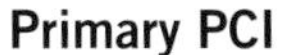

Primary PCI

Not every analysis supports the current strategy of directing patients with a suspected ACS to a tertiary care hospital with interventional facilities. For example the GRACE group looked prospectively at 28,825 ACS patients enrolled in 106 hospitals in 14 countries, 77% of whom were admitted to hospitals with cardiac catheterization facilities.[209] Not surprisingly the availability of a cath lab was associated with more frequent use of PCI (41% versus 3.9%) and coronary artery bypass surgery (7.1% versus 0.7%). After adjustment of baseline characteristics, the risk of death at 6 months was significantly higher (14%) in patients first admitted to centres with interventional facilities due to the risk of in-hospital bleeding complications and stroke. These authors argue that these findings support the current strategy of admitting ACS patients as rapidly as possible to the nearest hospital, irrespective of the availability of a cath lab, and argues against the early routine transport of these patients to a specialized regional centre with interventional facilities.

> *“Primary stenting is superior to balloon angioplasty alone”*

How does primary PCI compare with immediate thrombolysis in the management of acute MI? Dalby *et al*[210] performed a meta-analysis of six trials involving 3750 patients comparing primary angioplasty and thrombolysis. They found that the combined endpoint of death/reinfarction and stroke was significantly reduced by 42% in the group transferred for primary PCI compared with the group receiving on-site thrombolysis. When considered separately, reinfarction was reduced by 68% and stroke by 56% and there was a 19% trend towards reduction in all-cause mortality. These workers conclude that, even when transfer to an angioplasty centre is necessary, primary PCI remains superior to immediate thrombolysis. Even with such data the debate on whether moving away from first-line thrombolysis is appropriate or practical still continues.[211]

PCI options

Stents are now used in the majority of PCIs. Now drug-eluting stents, which elute an anti-proliferative agent reducing neointimal hyperplasia and the risk of re-stenosis without systemic toxicity, have become available (Figure 57). As these drug-eluting stents are considerably more expensive than bare metal stents their widespread use is more restricted.

Revascularization of STEMI patients with balloon angioplasty alone has been compared with primary stenting in several trials.[212,213] Reperfusion, reinfarction and mortality were similar with both techniques but primary stenting was associated with lower late target-vessel revascularization. With the advent of drug-eluting stents there

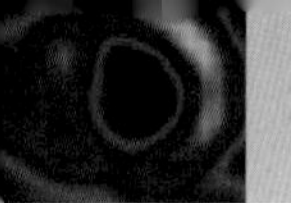

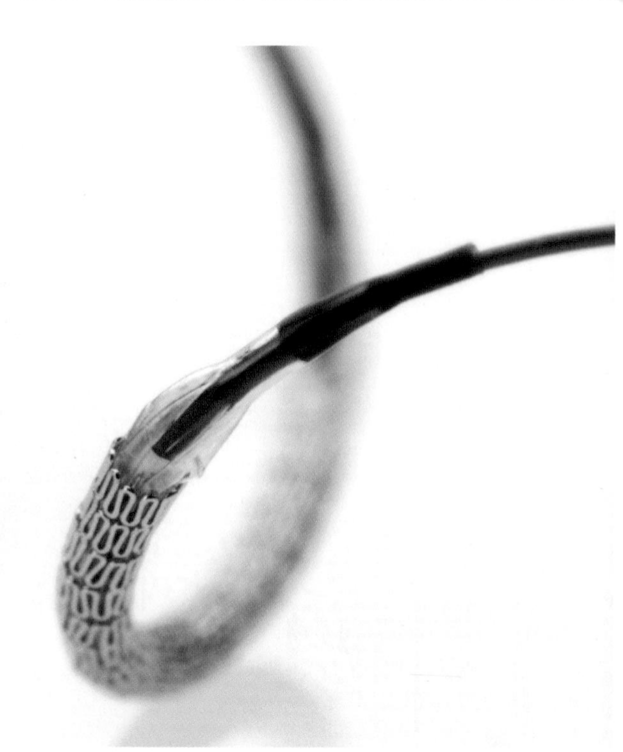

Fig. 57 Drug-eluting stent. The Endeavour ABT-578-coated cobalt alloy drug-eluting stent, shown with delivery system. Picture courtesy of Medtronic.

has been a marked reduction of in-stent restenosis. Both the rapamycin-coated stent and the paclitaxel-eluting stent have shown improved outcomes for elective PCI compared with bare metal stents.[214,215] Initial data using drug-eluting stents in acute MI demonstrate short-term patency and periprocedural safety similar to bare metal stents.[216]

Adjunctive medications with PCI

"Drug-eluting stents require prolonged administration of aspirin plus clopidogrel"

- **Antiplatelet drugs** Aspirin 81–325 mg/day is recommended for all tolerant patients, indefinitely. Clopidogrel 75 mg/day should be added for at least 4 weeks after stenting with a bare metal stent. Drug-eluting stents require longer clopidogrel treatment (sirolimus stents 3 months, paclitaxil stents 6 months). ESC guidelines[105] may differ slightly to those from the AHA/ACC, for example in patients where there is doubt about whether they are chronically pretreated or not a loading dose of aspirin 500 mg orally is recommended more than 3 hours pre-PCI, or 300 mg iv prior to the procedure. Similarly clopidogrel should be additionally administered with a loading dose of 600 mg. Clopidogrel should be administered in addition to aspirin for 6–12 months after a drug-eluting stent to avoid late vessel thrombosis.

Indication	Eptifibatide*	Abciximab	Tirofiban^
Elective PCI	180 g/kg and a second 180 g/kg bolus 10 minutes later followed by iv infusion of 2.0 g/kg/min for 18–24 hours after angiography[122]	0.25 mg/kg administered over 10–60 minutes before the start of PCI, followed by iv infusion of 0.125 g/kg/min (to a maximum of 10 g/min) for 12 hours[121]	10 g/kg followed by infusion of 0.15 g/kg/min for 18 to 24 hours[123]
Urgent/ emergency PCI	180 g/kg and a second 180 g/kg bolus 10 minutes later followed by iv infusion of 2.0 g/kg/min for 18–24 hours after angiography[203]	0.25 mg/kg administered over 10–60 minutes before the start of PCI, followed by iv infusion of 0.125 g/kg/min (to a maximum of 10 g/min) for 12 hours[205]	25 g/kg over 3 minutes, followed by an infusion of 0.15 g/kg/min for 18 to 24 hours (STRATEGY trial dose)[126]

* Patients with an estimated clearance (using the Cockroft-Gault equation) <50 mL/min or, if creatinine clearance is not available, a serum creatinine >2.0 mg/dL should receive half the usual rate of infusion

^ Patients with an estimated clearance (using the Cockroft-Gault equation) <30 mL/min should receive half the usual rate of infusion

Fig. 58 Dosing of GP IIb/IIIa inhibitors during PCI.

- **Heparin** Weight-adjusted UFH is started immediately for patients going for catheterization. The goal for aPTT is 50–70 seconds and monitoring should be undertaken 6-hourly to assess need for heparin dose adjustment.
- **GP IIb/IIIa inhibitors** There is conflicting evidence regarding the added benefit of GP IIb/IIIa during PCI for STEMI. The general recommendation is to use a GP IIb/IIIa inhibitor early. The 2004 ACC/AHA guidelines assign the GP IIb/IIIa agents a "2a recommendation" and the current data suggest an advantage with abciximab. Recent findings from the STRATEGY trial[126] suggest that tirofiban-supported sirolimus-eluting stenting holds promise for improving outcomes in acute MI patients undergoing primary PCI.
- **Warfarin** Full anticoagulation with warfarin is recommended for 1–3 months post STEMI for patients at high risk for emboli. High-risk patients include those with:
  - left ventricular thrombus
  - left ventricular aneurysm
  - left ventricular ejection fraction <30% in the absence of thrombus.

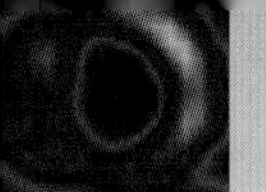

Management of complications of PCI

The most common complications of PCI include volume overload, dye-induced acute renal insufficiency, bleeding and groin complications (arterio-venous fistula, pseudoaneurysm, nerve compression and expanding haematoma). Haematocrit, blood urea nitrogen and creatinine should be obtained within 12 to 24 hours post procedure. A falling haematocrit often requires a bleeding evaluation with an abdominal CT scan to screen for retroperitoneal haematoma. Vascular ultrasound is indicated to assess a large groin haematoma, especially when there is a localized murmur over the access site.

Rescue PCI after failed thrombolysis for STEMI

“Coronary stenting after failed thrombolysis has been shown to be safe”

To obtain clinical benefit from reperfusion therapy patients must achieve optimal (TIMI grade 3) flow. Thrombolytic therapy alone fails to restore TIMI grade 3 flow in up to 54% of patients.[191,217] Non-resolving chest pain, lack of reduction of electrocardiographic ST elevation by >50%, and electrical or haemodynamic instability can be indicators of failed reperfusion. Salvage balloon angioplasty without stenting appears to have minimal added clinical benefit after failed fibrinolysis and is often complicated by excess bleeding complications.[218] Furthermore failed rescue balloon angioplasty is associated with increased mortality.[218,219]

In contrast coronary stenting after failed thrombolysis has been shown to be safe and enhance myocardial salvage compared with balloon-only rescue attempts but data are lacking for a mortality endpoint.[220,221] The REACT trial compared rescue PCI, repeat thrombolysis, or conservative care in patients with persistent ST elevation 90 minutes after fibrinolytic therapy.[221] Rescue PCI reduced death, reinfarction and heart failure compared with the other strategies. When possible, rescue stenting is recommended for failed thrombolysis. The major concerns regarding rescue stenting are:

1. Identifying failed thrombolysis early enough to preserve any myocardium.
2. Increased risk of major bleeding when adding a GP IIb/IIIa inhibitor while a fibrinolytic drug is still active.

Management of no-reflow phenomenon and residual intracoronary thrombus

As described previously (pages 80–85), the establishment of infarct-related artery patency may have severely reduced myocardial perfusion due to either microvascular obstruction or reperfusion injury. Incomplete (<50%) resolution of ST elevation following PCI is a marker of microvascular obstruction.[222] Several strategies have

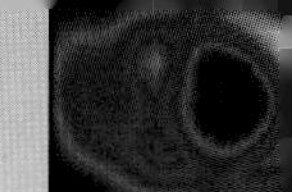

been assessed in an attempt to enhance distal perfusion. GP IIb/IIIa receptor blockers inhibit platelet/fibrin thrombus formation and reduce distal microvascular obstruction. These drugs have established benefit especially in the setting of stent placement. Adenosine has a potential multifaceted benefit reducing localized coronary spasm, inhibiting leukocyte-induced endothelial dysfunction with lowered pro-oxidant stress, cytokine release and apoptosis. The AMISTAD II trial randomized patients starting 15 minutes post primary angioplasty to adenosine 50–70 μg/kg/minute versus placebo for 3 hours.[223] Adenosine-treated patients had smaller infarct size ($p<0.05$) and a trend towards less heart failure and lower mortality. Verapamil may reduce microvascular spasm and platelet aggregation but adequate clinical trials to support its benefit are lacking. Nicorandil, a hybrid nitrate and potassium channel opener, is a potent vasodilator with possible anti-inflammatory properties. Small clinical studies have suggested that nicorandil reduces the incidence of "no reflow", improves left ventricular function and enhances recovery of ST-segment elevation.[224,225] A large double-blind placebo-controlled trial is in progress. Results of intervention with other pharmacologic agents including anti-neutrophil drugs (CD 18 antibody), complement inhibitors (pexelizumab), glucose-insulin-potassium and sodium-hydrogen exchange inhibitors (cariporide) have been either negative or mixed.

Distal protection and clot extraction devices are attractive mechanical approaches to enhance flow and reduce microvascular embolization. Thus far however, no study has shown superior clinical outcome with any particular product, but there is hope with future trials using modified devices.

Other treatments and special clinical settings

Emergency coronary bypass surgery

Consideration of acute surgical reperfusion is rarely needed with the current availability of thrombolysis and PCI. Emergency CABG surgery may be beneficial but has an attendant higher mortality compared with elective surgery (6.4% versus 2.0%, excluding patients with cardiogenic shock).[226] Emergency CABG should be reserved for patients with ongoing ischaemia, or haemodynamic or electrical instability who are not candidates for PCI or fibrinolysis, or have failed PCI. These patients should have extensive myocardium at risk with either severe left main or multivessel disease amenable to revascularization. Selected patients <75 years old who develop cardiogenic shock within <36 hours from onset of STEMI may benefit from surgery if performed within 18 hours of shock.

"Emergency coronary bypass surgery is recommended for unstable patients who are not candidates for fibrinolysis or PCI, or have failed PCI"

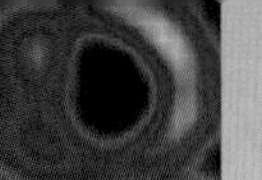

“IABP may be utilized to stabilize patients with large infarcts and severely impaired coronary perfusion prior to PCI or coronary bypass surgery”

Intra-aortic balloon pumping (IABP)

IABP insertion is used to stabilize patients with large infarctions, borderline coronary perfusion and/or haemodynamic compromise. Though IABP can be beneficial, balloon pumping alone does not usually reduce mortality. Rather this intervention may be helpful to stabilize patients prior to PCI or surgical revascularization. Criteria for IABP are:

- systolic blood pressure <90 mmHg
- low cardiac output or cardiogenic shock
- refractory chest pain or haemodynamic instability
- refractory polymorphic ventricular tachycardia
- refractory pulmonary congestion.

Reperfusion in the elderly

The preferred treatment strategy for STEMI in the elderly has not been systematically studied. Review of existing data suggests a net benefit from fibrinolysis for patients over 75 years old.[227] It should be recognized however that the risk of intracranial haemorrhage increases with age, possibly more so with the fibrin-specific agents. Data from the ASSENT-3 trial suggest a regimen of tenecteplase with weight-based heparin.[197] Comparing PCI versus medical treatment with fibrinolysis, both randomized clinical trials and observational studies suggest that PCI results in lower mortality than thrombolysis in the elderly.[228] At present a recommended strategy is rapid primary PCI (chest pain triage-to-balloon time <90 minutes) if available within 12 hours of ischaemic symptoms. If PCI is not available, treatment should comprise a fibrinolytic with weight-adjusted heparin. A GP IIb/IIIa antagonist is recommended as an adjunct to PCI but not with thrombolysis.

“PCI is the preferred treatment for patients with cardiogenic shock”

Cardiogenic shock and CHF

“Patients with cardiogenic shock can benefit from PCI within 36 hours from the onset of STEMI if shock has persisted less than 18 hours”

IABP is of limited benefit but may be a helpful bridge to revascularization. Early PCI has been shown to be beneficial compared with thrombolysis. The SHOCK trial was a randomized clinical trial that compared the strategy of medical stabilization versus emergency revascularization (PCI or coronary bypass surgery) for patients with hypotension secondary to STEMI.[229] Mortality at 6 months, though high as expected for this condition, was significantly lower in the revascularization group versus the medically treated group (50.3% versus 63.1%, $p<0.027$). The desired time frame for PCI is within 36 hours of STEMI onset and within 18 hours of the onset of shock. PCI can still be helpful for patients with severe CHF who are within 12 hours of symptom onset. Though the benefit in the randomized

1. How much time has elapsed since chest pain onset?

2. What is the risk of mortality?

Checklist for STEMI treatment

3. What is the risk of bleeding? Is there:
a. History of intracranial haemorrhage?
b. >4% risk of intracranial haemorrhage?
c. Closed head or facial trauma within 3 months?
d. Uncontrolled hypertension?
e. Ischaemic stroke within past 3 months?

4. What is the availability of PCI?
a. How much time to activate cardiac catheterization laboratory?
b. How long to transport and effect PCI? (PCI delay beyond 1 hour reduces the advantage over immediate fibrin-specific fibrinolytics especially when symptoms are <3 hours' duration).

Fig. 59 Checklist to determine optimal strategy for treatment of STEMI.

Emergency Department treatment

Aspirin 162–325 mg by mouth (European doses available as aspirin 150–300 mg)

Weight-based UFH or LMWH (selected patients)

Full-dose tenecteplase, alteplase, reteplase or streptokinase (door-to-needle time <30 minutes)

(*alternative consideration for transfer to hospital with catheterization services – see below)

Coronary Care Unit

Glyceryl trinitrate (either intravenous, by mouth or transdermal)

Morphine sulphate (as required for pain)

Beta-blockers (when stable)

ACE inhibitors (especially if anterior MI, CHF)

Statin therapy

Transfer to hospital with cardiac catheterization services

* Withhold fibrinolysis and transfer if patient can undergo catheterization within 90 minutes
* If transfer and catheterization cannot be performed within 90 minutes, administer fibrinolysis and consider transfer to catheterization centre later

Fig. 60 Algorithm for sites without interventional services.

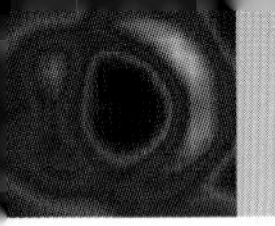

Fig. 61
Recommendations for reperfusion: fibrinolysis versus PCI.

Presentation	Situation	Recommendation
Early presentation (within 3 hours of symptom onset)	PCI available quickly (door-to-balloon <90 minutes)	Either fibrinolysis or PCI
	PCI available but delayed (door-to-balloon >90 minutes)	Fibrinolysis preferred
	PCI not readily available	Fibrinolysis preferred
	High-risk STEMI (cardiogenic shock or Killip class 3–4)	PCI preferred
	Contraindications to fibrinolysis	PCI preferred
	Diagnosis of STEMI questionable	Bedside echo and/or catheterization may be needed to determine need for reperfusion

Presentation	Recommendation
Late presentation (over 3 hours from symptom onset)	Can consider thrombolysis even as late as 12 hours but improvement will be marginal and outcome is better with PCI
	There may be benefit 12–24 hours beyond chest pain onset if symptoms are persistent
	Asymptomatic patients usually derive benefit from reperfusion if >12 hours from symptom onset

SHOCK patients was limited to patients <75 years old, elderly patients in the non-randomized SHOCK registry had marked mortality reduction with revascularization compared with medical treatment alone or delayed revascularization.[230]

Summary guidelines

Triage and treatment of patients with STEMI is summarized in Figure 63. Patients should be rapidly categorized by:

- duration of symptoms
- availablity of PCI (including both time to transfer patient to catheterization capable facility and time to mobilize the catheterization team)
- contraindications to thrombolytics
- hypotension.

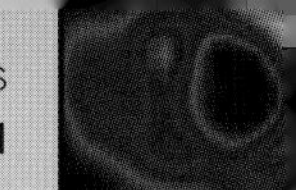

Emergency Department treatment

Aspirin 162–325 mg by mouth (European doses available as aspirin 150–300 mg)

UFH or enoxaparin

Cardiac Catheterization Laboratory

PCI

- Abciximab (alternative eptifbatide)
- Clopidogrel 300 mg loading dose – If CABG required rather than PCI then withhold clopidogrel
- Continue aspirin and heparin (LMWH or UFH)

Fig. 62 Algorithm for sites with interventional cardiac services.

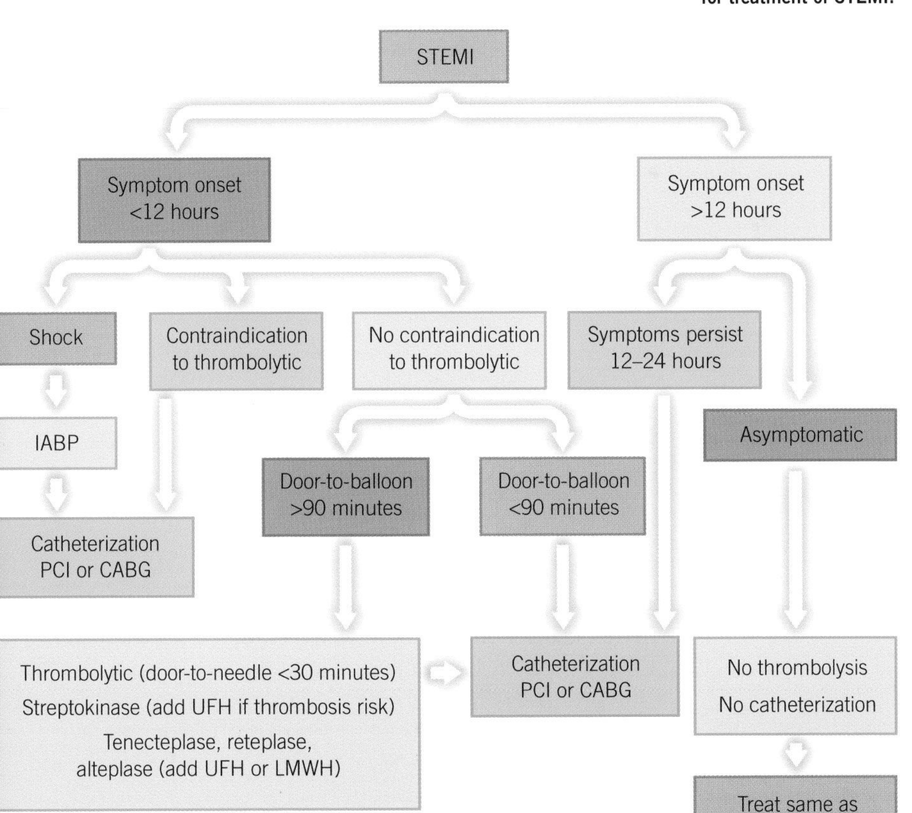

Fig. 63 Flow diagram for treatment of STEMI.

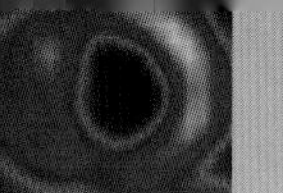

Special populations

The elderly

"In the Western World there is an ageing population"

Life-expectancy is increasing dramatically in the UK, where women can expect to live well over 80 years and men more than 75 years (the rates in the US are almost identical). At present about 18% of the UK population is over 65 years of age and in 25 years time this will become one in four individuals. Cardiovascular diseases occur predominantly among older people and are the leading cause of death in both men and women above 65 years of age.[231] We are now seeing an increasing incidence of angina (about 3.6% per annum)[232] and heart failure (median age of first presentation around 76 years, commonly secondary to CAD). Patients aged over 75 years now constitute about 10% of ACS. Secondary prevention may be implemented with considerable benefit and little increase in risk for many elderly patients.[233] Randomized controlled studies in ACS, on the whole, have actively excluded the very elderly (i.e. those over 80 years), subjects with significant co-morbidity or those receiving polypharmacy. In addition, variability in the definition of "elderly" hinders comparisons between studies.

Risk factors and presentation

"ACS are common in the elderly and associated with poorer outcomes"

The risk factor profile for CHD varies with age; in patients presenting with acute STEMI there are nearly three times as many women with almost double the prevalence of hypertension and diabetes in those ≥70 years of age as compared with the ≤49 years age group (Figure 64).[234]

Atypical presentation of ACS in the elderly, for example confusion, dyspnoea or neurological symptoms, may result in delayed diagnosis and initiation of definitive treatment. Complications are more common post acute MI, including atrial fibrillation, cardiac failure, conduction abnormalities, stroke and mechanical complications such as ventricular rupture, which undoubtedly impact on the higher mortality.[235]

Treatment options in the elderly

Medical therapy

Reduced renal drug clearance and hepatic metabolism and an increase in target organ sensitivity due to changes in pharmacokinetics and pharmacodynamics may result in a higher drug plasma concentration and thus an increased frequency of adverse effects in the elderly. Drug interactions are common due to multiple co-morbidities and polypharmacy. A national survey of over-65-year-olds in the US revealed that over 40% used five or more different medications each week and 12% used ≥10 per week.[236] In younger patients presenting with ACS standard care may result in the addition of five new drugs. While these

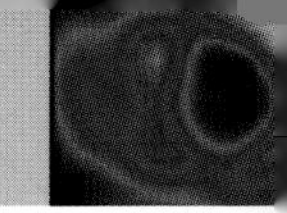

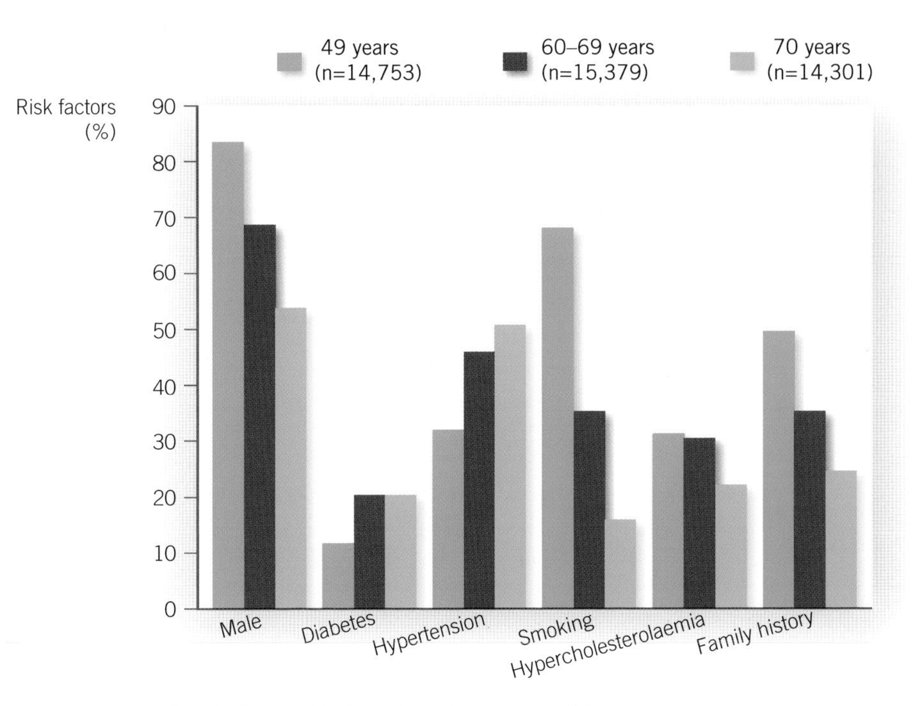

Fig. 64 Percentage of initial uncomplicated MI patients with various cardiac risk factors stratified by age group. Data from the Second National Registry of Myocardial Infarction.[234]

drugs are generally of value in elderly patients it seems sensible to tailor precise treatment to the individual taking into consideration co-morbidity, current therapy, general health, cognitive function and life-expectancy. Vigilance for undue side effects of treatment is necessary.

Despite a higher risk profile, patients aged over 75 years presenting with UA/NSTEMI are treated less aggressively with medical therapy and interventions than their younger counterparts.

- *Antiplatelet treatment* Aspirin has been shown to reduce mortality after STEMI in a wide spectrum of age groups. Yet older patients, often with higher risk characteristics, do not commonly receive it. Reduced prescribing of aspirin is in part due to the fear of aspirin-induced gastritis, although this has not been confirmed in studies.[237] Anecdotally many elderly patients declare an allergy to aspirin when truly they have experienced dyspeptic symptoms. In summary, aspirin, unless truly contraindicated, should be used in all elderly patients with STEMI or UA/NSTEMI.

  Clopidogrel is generally prescribed in addition to aspirin in patients presenting with NSTEMI. Recent data also suggest a benefit in STEMI,[164] although patients over 75 years were excluded and as such there is no evidence in this group. A recent population-based study confirmed a small overall risk (hospitalization rates for bleeding 0.03 per patient-year with aspirin alone

“Polypharmacy and co-morbidities are common”

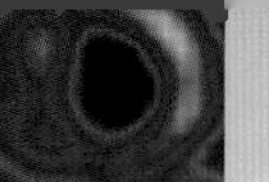

versus 0.07 per patient-year for aspirin and clopidogrel combination).[238] As such in higher-risk elderly patients presenting with NSTEMI it seems reasonable to add in clopidogrel but perhaps this should be for a relatively short duration (e.g. 2–3 months).

"Altered pharmacokinetics may increase the risk of drug side effects"

- *Beta-blockers* The ACC/AHA guidelines recommend the prompt administration of beta-blockers in all patients without contra-indications post STEMI[155] and in patients presenting with UA/NSTEMI.[133]

  In one observational database analysis of over 200,000 Medicare beneficiaries post acute MI only 34% of patients received beta-blockers on discharge.[239] Numbers were lowest in the very elderly, blacks, patients with heart failure, low ejection fractions, chronic obstructive pulmonary disease (COPD), elevated serum creatinine level, or type 1 diabetes mellitus. Beta-blocker treatment was associated with a 40% reduction in 2-year mortality and a benefit was seen in all subgroups of patients treated with beta-blockers compared with the untreated group (32% mortality reduction in the over-80-year-olds and 40% in patients with COPD).

  The reluctance to prescribe beta-blockers in the elderly is probably due to increased co-morbidity in this age group, in particular COPD and peripheral vascular disease. One study reported a similar survival benefit with beta-blocker therapy following MI in elderly patients with mild COPD/asthma not requiring beta-agonists compared with patients without chronic lung disease.[240]
- *Other anti-ischaemic drugs* Calcium antagonists are recommended when refractory symptoms are present, for control of hypertension (despite beta-blockade and ACE inhibitors) or for patients who have a genuine contraindication to beta-blockade (rate limiting drug). In the elderly, nitrates and calcium antagonists tend to be associated with a higher incidence of postural hypotension.

"Drugs deemed beneficial in younger patients are in general perceived to be of value in the elderly"

- *ACE inhibitors* According to the ACC/AHA guidelines, the use of ACE inhibitors in the elderly post STEMI should be limited to those patients with cardiac failure, reduced LV ejection fraction or previous MI.[155]

  A meta-analysis of four placebo-controlled clinical trials (n=100,000) post acute MI demonstrated a 10.8% 30-day mortality reduction in patients aged 65–74 years treated with ACE inhibitors. The percentage of patients aged >75 years varied from 9% in CCS-1 to 23% in CONSENSUS-II. Hypotension and renal dysfunction with ACE inhibitor therapy were more common in patients over 75 years of age and there was no evidence of any significant survival benefit in this patient group.[241]

In UA/NSTEMI most would agree that ACE inhibitors should be used in elderly patients with hypertension, LV dysfunction or clinical heart failure, and high-risk diabetic patients.

- *Lipid-lowering therapy* Large randomized trials have consistently demonstrated that cholesterol-lowering therapy in patients of all ages with established CHD provides a significant mortality benefit.[242,243] However there is a decreased rate of prescribing in the elderly due to the concerns about side effects in frail patients with multiple co-morbidities.[235] Predicted life-expectancy may contribute to under utilization of statins. It is important to note that statins have early benefits on outcomes independent of lipid-lowering properties. If life-expectancy is >12 months then reduction in lipids may also provide benefit.
- *Anticoagulants* A meta-analysis demonstrated that subcutaneous enoxaparin (LMWH) use was associated with a 20% reduction in death and serious cardiac ischaemic events when compared with standard UFH iv infusion in patients with UA/NSTEMI (n=7081, mean age 64–65 years).[244] The treatment benefit was observed at day 2 and continued until day 43. This was at the expense of an increase in the rate of minor haemorrhage with enoxaparin.

  Anticoagulants should however be used with caution in the very elderly as the risk of bleeding may be higher due to general frailty, multiple falls and co-morbidity. Weights should not be estimated. When considering LMWH the presence of significant renal impairment should be excluded (ideally by estimated glomerular filtration rate since in the elderly loss of muscle mass may give false reassurance if using serum creatinine); if present a reduction in dose or avoidance of LMWH altogether is suggested. When using UFH a weight-based bolus and infusion is recommended in older patients in order to avoid bleeding complications.[235,245]

  It is the authors' opinion that in the very elderly (>80 years old) LMWH should not be routinely prescribed for prolonged periods (e.g. >48 hours) in UA/NSTEMI unless there are ongoing symptoms or particularly high-risk features.

- *Thrombolytics* The efficacy of thrombolytic therapy in the elderly remains uncertain. The ACC/AHA guidelines recommend thrombolysis in patients who present to hospital within 12 hours of symptom onset with either ST elevation or new left bundle branch block on ECG without contraindications (age not specified). The evidence for the benefit of thrombolysis has been well established in younger patients but is not as conclusive in the over-75-year age group.[155,246]

  The GUSTO-1 trial compared various thrombolytic regimens in different age groups.[247] It found that alteplase in combination

“Despite higher risk in the elderly, PCI, when readily available, is preferred over pharmacologic reperfusion”

“Thrombolysis plus weight-adjusted heparin should be considered when early PCI is not available”

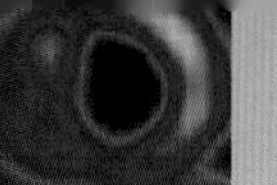

with aspirin and heparin was associated with an increased risk of intracranial haemorrhage in patients over 75 years (2.1%) versus the under-75-year-olds (0.5%). There was no increased risk of stroke in older ages with streptokinase in GUSTO-1.

"Fibrinolysis can benefit patients over 75 years old but carries an increased risk of intracranial haemorrhage"

Thiemann *et al*[248] found an insignificant reduction in 30-day mortality with thrombolysis among patients aged 65–75 years and a significant increase in mortality in the over-75-years group (hazard ratio 1.38, p=0.003). Similarly another study of 2659 patients aged over 65 years who received thrombolytic therapy for acute MI reported a diminished benefit with increasing age and it was found to be detrimental among patients aged over 80 years.[249]

In other studies[250,251] it has been demonstrated that, although thrombolysis was not significantly associated with a lower in-hospital mortality in the older age groups, there was a mortality benefit seen at 1 year (Berger *et al*) and 18 months (Gitt *et al*).

Despite limited data the current consensus is to consider treatment of elderly patients who present early (<12 hours) with thrombolytics plus weight-adjusted heparin. Patients at high risk for intracranial haemorrhage should be excluded from pharmacologic reperfusion.

PCI

"PCI is the preferred treatment for patients with cardiogenic shock"

- *Primary PCI versus thrombolysis* Given the increased risk of bleeding complications with thrombolysis in the elderly, primary PCI, where available might be considered the preferred treatment for this age group. A database analysis of over 20,000 elderly patients (average age 73 ± 6 years) post acute MI compared the outcomes of primary PCI versus thrombolysis. Patients undergoing primary PCI had a significantly lower 30-day (8.7% versus 11.9%, p=0.001) and 1-year mortality (14.4% versus 17.6%, p=0.001).[252] Furthermore, the incidence of post-MI angina, reinfarction, cerebral haemorrhage, stroke and major bleeding was significantly higher in the group receiving thrombolysis.

  Data from an observational registry of 2975 elderly patients aged ≥70 years eligible for reperfusion therapy post acute STEMI revealed that 12.7% underwent primary PCI and 26.7% received thrombolysis. After adjustment for baseline differences, patients receiving primary PCI showed a lower rate of reinfarction (1.1% versus 5.7%, OR 0.15, 95% CI 0.05–0.44) and mortality (13.5% versus 14.8%, OR 0.62, 95% CI 0.39–0.96).[253]

"PCI results in lower mortality than fibrinolysis in the elderly"

  Despite the benefit of primary PCI in elderly patients post acute MI, there is a significant increase in morbidity and mortality seen in this age group when compared with younger patients. In a pooled analysis of over 3000 patients with acute MI treated with primary angioplasty in-hospital mortality was 10.2% in the ≥75-year-olds versus 1.8% in the younger patients.[254] However, given the even greater morbidity and mortality with thrombolysis, interventional cardiologists are often willing to take on these high-risk cases.

- *PCI and cardiogenic shock* The SHOCK trial randomized 302 patients with cardiogenic shock post acute MI to either early revascularization (PCI or CABG) or intensive medical therapy (including thrombolysis). A significantly lower mortality was seen in patients <75 years of age treated with early invasive therapy. On the contrary, patients over 75 years of age had higher 30-day, 6-month and 1-year mortality with early invasive therapy (75%, 79.2%, 79.2%, respectively) compared with intensive medical therapy (53.1%, 56.3%, 65.6%, respectively).[255] Though the benefit in the *randomized* SHOCK patients was limited to patients <75 years old, elderly patients in the *non-randomized* SHOCK registry had marked mortality reduction with revascularization compared with medical treatment alone or delayed revascularization.[230]
- *PCI versus CABG* A careful assessment of risks and benefits should be carried out in the elderly prior to consideration for surgery. CABG in the elderly is associated with an increased risk of mortality,[256] peri-operative stroke[257] and neurocognitive decline.[258]

  A pooled analysis of nearly 230,000 patients aged ≥75 years undergoing PCI and CABG in the US from 1991 to 1999 looked at revascularization risks and outcomes. Patients aged ≥75 years constitute a substantial percentage of patients undergoing revascularization, with a 10% increase being seen in the last decade. While procedural complications increase with age, the mortality following PCI and CABG was modest at 3% and 5.9%, respectively. In the CABG group mortality rates increased approximately 2% per decade to age 85 and then significantly increased to 10% after age 85. The most powerful predictors of in-hospital mortality in PCI were emergent case, shock and acute MI. In the case of CABG, the best single predictor of in-hospital mortality was prior surgery.[259]

> *"Management should be individualized and consider general and cognitive health, co-morbidity and life-expectancy"*

Gender and ethnic differences

Excessive rates of cardiovascular diseases are well recognized in various ethnic populations. These include Southern Asians from India, Pakistan, Bangladesh and Sri Lanka who emigrate to Europe and other Western countries. The prevalence of CHD is also extremely high within these Southern Asian countries.[260] Disparities in cardiovascular disease and related risk factors are also pervasive in the US, where life-expectancy remains higher in women than men and higher in whites than blacks by about 5 years.[261] African Caribbean patients in the UK have a significantly lower (by about one half) CHD risk compared with the majority of the population, however their risk of stroke is 1.5 to 2.5 times higher.[260] Stroke rates are also very high among African Americans and recent reports suggest that with acculturation CHD rates are increasing also. The US population has become ethnically diverse with the Hispanic segment becoming the fastest growing and currently representing 14–15% of the population and people of African descent representing another 12%. The Cardiovascular Science and Health Care Disparities Minority Health Summit has therefore recently published recommendations for action on the issue of racial/ethnic disparities at all levels of the medical care system.[262]

> *"Population registries and epidemiological surveys show differences (variations) in the incidence, and possibly clinical outcomes, in ACS among ethnic groups and female, compared with male, patients"*

The need for such recommendations, embracing research, advocacy and education, is underlined by findings from CRUSADE.[263] Using data from 400 American hospitals CRUSADE showed that black patients with NSTEMI ACS were less likely than whites to receive many evidence-based treatments, particularly those that are costly or newer. In TACTICS-TIMI-18,[264] after adjustment for baseline characteristics, non-white patients had a significantly worse prognosis than white patients, regardless of treatment approach. Although all patients had similar rates of angiography and revascularization there were lower rates of "non-protocol-guided therapies" including lower use of cardiac medications and coronary stenting during PCI in non-white patients. This has led to a call for better adherence to accepted guidelines to ensure that the best possible care is delivered to all patients regardless of race. Greater symptoms and functional impairment has also been observed in a prospective cohort of just under 2000 white and black patients, which showed that differential use of coronary revascularization may contribute to the poorer functional outcomes seen among black patients with documented CHD.[265]

> *"It is unknown to what extent variation relates to environmental, nutritional and lifestyle, as opposed to genetic, factors"*

While CHD and stroke are inversely related to education, income and poverty status,[261] ethnic differences in the presence of coronary calcification, homocysteine and Lp(a) lipoprotein (specific markers of atherosclerosis) may also play an important role in explaining outcomes among different ethnic groups. Some of these factors, including insulin resistance (and frequently diabetes) and increased markers of inflammation, such as CRP, are associated with central adiposity, which can lead to chronic endothelial dysfunction, and are favoured to explain excess risk among Asians.[260,266] Another factor however, is that coronary vessels are smaller in Southern Asians relative to Europeans, which increases technical difficulties during revascularization. Similarly, Asian patients frequently present with more diffuse atherosclerotic disease as is commonly seen angiographically in diabetes.

Smaller vessel size is also cited as one reason to explain why women with CHD have a worse prognosis than men. CHD has long been the

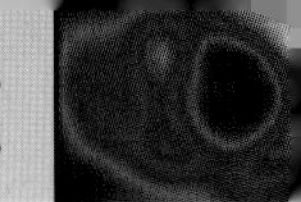

leading cause of morbidity and mortality in the US and other developed countries, and more women die from heart disease each year than from breast, ovarian and uterine cancer combined. There are gender-related differences in the pathophysiology of CHD, its presentation, diagnosis and response to treatments. Women tend to be older and have a greater risk profile at presentation. Differences in the perception and type of symptoms of ACS have been reported,[267] as well as lower diagnostic accuracy of non-invasive testing in women compared with men.[268] Differential expression of cardiac biomarkers by gender in patients with UA/NSTEMI has also been observed with women more likely to have elevated CRP and BNP, whereas men were more likely to have elevated troponins and CK-MB.[269] Despite presenting with higher risk characteristics and having higher in-hospital risk, women with ACS are treated less aggressively than men.[270] In addition women experience greater delays to intervention and are referred for diagnostic catheterization less frequently than are men.[271] While current evidence fails to show cardiac protection with hormone replacement therapy (HRT), control of conventional coronary risk factors provides comparable cardioprotection for men and women.[271] Further, recommendations contained in current guidelines are indeed "gender-neutral", while there are pervasive and continuing disparities in their application.

"Disparities and underutilization of diagnostic investigations and treatments have been identified in both situations"

Findings from the Singapore Myocardial Infarction Register (SMIR) have shown a higher incidence of acute MI among Indians and Malays compared with Chinese living in the city-state of Singapore. More recently, gender differences, with increased vulnerability in women among these groups, has been reported.[272] While not fully explained, this may in part be due to a selection bias of the most severe patients or to a delay in diagnosis. Current evidence suggests that increased use of therapeutic and interventional management strategies, including coronary stenting and CABG surgery, has favourably altered prognosis in women (women tend to fare as well as men and perhaps better after bypass surgery) particularly when data are adjusted for baseline characteristics.[271,273]

"Evidence suggests that greater efforts for prevention at both a primary and secondary level are required and that reshaping practice patterns (offering the same treatments) may dramatically improve outcomes in all patient groups"

Lanza[274] has further highlighted the complexities, suggesting that ethnic variations in the incidence and possible clinical outcome of acute CHD events "probably exist" but the causes of such differences are multiple. While environmental, nutritional, socioeconomic, cultural and lifestyle factors are likely to play a major role, genetic factors might significantly contribute also. Not all studies agree that ethnicity *per se* is an independent cardiovascular risk factor.[275]

The practical message therefore seems to be that, regardless of ethnicity or gender, patients with ACS should receive the same investigations and evidence-based treatments regardless of where they present or reside.

Prevention of heart disease and acute events

Preventing heart disease remains a public health priority. Control of cardiovascular risk factors is needed in high-risk populations (primary prevention) and aggressive lifestyle and pharmacological interventions are warranted in those with established disease. This section provides the evidence on which international recommendations for primary and secondary CHD prevention are based.

Cardiovascular risk factors

The INTERHEART study,[276] a large standardized case-control study of acute MI in 52 countries, clearly showed that conventional cardiovascular risk factors, such as abnormal lipids, smoking, hypertension and so forth, account for "an overwhelming large proportion" (>90%) of the risk of an initial heart attack. That is not to say that other novel risk factors such as raised levels of CRP and homocysteine are not important amplifiers of the disease. CHD mortality rates have been declining in the US, the UK and other developed countries since the 1970s. Between 1981 and 2000 CHD deaths in England and Wales decreased by 62% in men and 45% in women in the 25–84 year age range. Over half of the mortality decline has been attributed to population risk factor reductions,[277] particularly smoking; and more than 40% is attributable to treatments in individuals (about 11% from secondary prevention).

"Lipid modifying therapy provides early (less than a year) benefits in high- and moderate-risk individuals without signs or symptoms of CHD"

Smoking

Cigarette smoking is one of the most important modifiable risk factors for CHD.[278] Smoking adversely affects endothelial function. Smoking-enhanced platelet aggregation and platelet thrombus formation are important mechanisms for the increased risk of acute coronary events in smokers. A recent prospective cohort study of 967 CHD patients[279] has confirmed that major beneficial effects are expected within the first year of smoking cessation after acute manifestation of CHD.

Diet and lipid modifying therapy

Diet also plays a key role in both primary and secondary CHD prevention. The Mediterranean diet is low in saturated fat and high in unsaturated fats, especially olive oil, and has been shown to increase survival in older people[280] as well as to reduce cardiac death and reinfarction rates in heart attack survivors. A diet low in saturated fats is the major lifestyle change necessary to decrease LDL cholesterol. Responses to dietary modification are however highly variable and lipid lowering drugs will be needed for primary prevention in high-risk individuals and for most patients with CHD. Data from epidemiological studies and clinical trials have shown that for every 1 mg/dL (0.025 mmol/L) reduction in LDL cholesterol the relative risk of CHD is reduced by 1% (Figure 65).[281] These benefits extend to LDL cholesterol levels of 50–60 mg/dL (1.3–1.5 mmol/L), well below the previously recommended target of 100 mg/dL (2.5 mmol/L) for high-risk patients.

"Benefits are seen in young and older patients, males and females, with both high and "average" baseline cholesterol values"

Lipid lowering therapy unequivocally reduces morbidity and mortality. The earlier HMG-CoA reductase inhibitors (statins), such as simvastatin, lower total cholesterol by around 30% or more and reduce cardiovascular endpoints by a similar percentage. Such findings support the view that statin therapy stabilizes lipid-rich atherosclerotic plaques of mild-to-moderate severity and therefore makes them less vulnerable to rupture. Statins also appear to exert anti-inflammatory and anti-thrombotic effects, referred to as pleiotropic effects, and may modulate endothelial dysfunction independently of their lipid lowering.

The newest generation of statins, such as atorvastatin and rosuvastatin, can reduce total cholesterol by more than 60%, but there are no outcome data yet with the latter agent.

There are three principal placebo-controlled trials of statin therapy in primary prevention of CHD. The WOSCOPS trial[282] evaluated pravastatin 40 mg and placebo in 6595 high-risk middle-aged men with a mean plasma cholesterol of 7.0 mmol/L (272 mg/dL) and a fasting LDL cholesterol of at least 4.0 mmol/L. After 5 years the statin lowered LDL cholesterol by 26% and reduced the primary endpoint of non-fatal MI or CHD death by 31%. Total mortality was lowered 22% without any increase in non-cardiovascular deaths. The principal message was that pravastatin treatment resulted in impressive reductions in CHD among men with moderate hypercholesterolaemia and no history of MI. A *post hoc* analysis also showed that pravastatin therapy reduced the risk of developing diabetes by 30% in the WOSCOPS trial.

"Statin treatment reduces total, all-cause and cardiovascular mortality in patients with established CHD"

AFCAPS/TexCAPS[283] compared lovastatin 20–40 mg/day with placebo for prevention of the first acute major coronary event in 6605 healthy men and women without clinically evident CHD and average total cholesterol (mean 5.71 mmol/L; 221 mg/dL) and LDL cholesterol (3.9 mmol/L; 150 mg/dL) but with low levels of HDL cholesterol (0.94 mmol/L; 36 mg/dL). After an average follow-up of 5.2 years, treatment reduced LDL cholesterol by 25% and HDL cholesterol was raised by 6%. The primary endpoint, composed of fatal and non-fatal MI, UA and sudden cardiac death, was significantly reduced by 37% with lovastatin. Secondary endpoints such as UA and revascularization procedures were also significantly reduced by 34% and 33%, respectively. Treatment benefits were consistent in both men and women, the elderly, hypertensives and smokers. This important study is

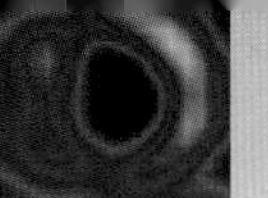

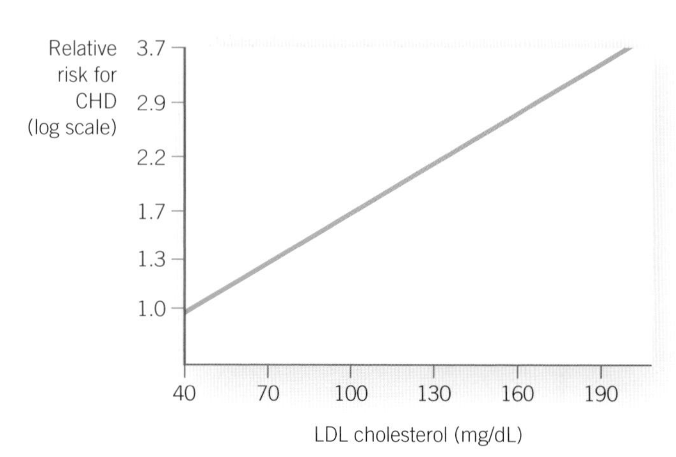

Fig. 65 Relative risk for CHD versus LDL cholesterol. Reproduced with permission from Grundy SM, Cleeman JI, Merz CNB, et al. Implications of recent clinical trials for the National Cholesterol Education Program Adult Treatment Panel III Guidelines. Circulation 2004;110:227–239.

complementary to WOSCOPS, extending the evidence base for primary prevention of CHD.

More recently ASCOT-LLA[284] assessed cholesterol lowering in the primary prevention of CHD in hypertensive patients who are not conventionally deemed dyslipidaemic. Conducted in 1035 individuals with a non-fasting total cholesterol of 6.5 mmol/L (251 mg/dL) or less who were randomized to atorvastatin 10 mg/day or placebo, the trial was planned for a 5-year follow-up but was terminated early at a median follow-up of 3.3 years. There was a 36% relative risk reduction in the primary endpoint, non-fatal MI and CHD death, associated with atorvastatin treatment. This benefit emerged in the first year of follow-up. Fatal and non-fatal stroke were also reduced significantly by 27%. This early divergence of the survival curves was also seen in the other two primary prevention trials.

Figure 66 shows the relationship between LDL cholesterol and CHD event rates in the key primary prevention trials.[285]

“Benefits extend to those with low initial LDL cholesterol”

Earlier key trials of secondary prevention such as 4S,[286] CARE[243] and LIPID[287] together enrolled almost 18,000 men and women with a history of MI and/or angina. These trials along with the largest statin trial, the Heart Protection Study (HPS),[288] which enrolled over 20,500 patients, have become the “gold standard” in terms of event reduction. In these trials, which had follow-up periods of 5 to 6 years, LDL cholesterol reductions ranged between 25 and 32%, and these were associated with reductions in total mortality between 13 and 30% and reductions in cardiovascular endpoints between 5.4 and 34%. These findings were remarkably consistent despite the fact that baseline total cholesterol fell within the upper range of Western populations in 4S (4.9 mmol/L; 190 mg/dL) to only average values in CARE (3.6

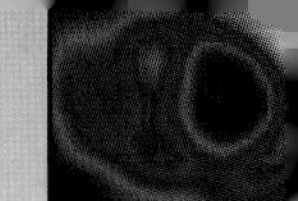

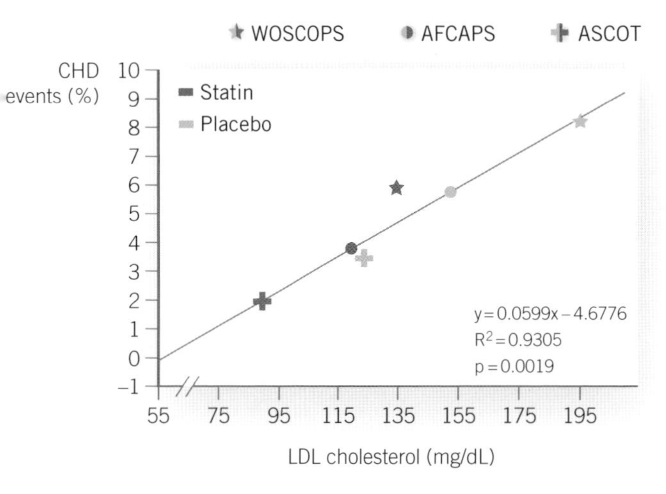

Fig. 66 CHD events versus LDL cholesterol – primary prevention trials. Reproduced with permission from O'Keefe JH, Cordain L, Harris WH, et al. Optimal low-density lipoprotein is 50 to 70 mg/dl. Lower is better and physiologically normal. J Am Coll Cardiol 2004;43:2142–2146. © Elsevier

mmol/L; 139 mg/dL) and covered a broad spectrum in LIPID (median 3.9 mmol/L; 150 mg/dL). HPS enrolled patients with a wide range of baseline LDL cholesterol ≥3.5 mmol/L (135 mg/dL) and established that there is no threshold LDL cholesterol below which therapy should not be initiated: for example reducing LDL cholesterol from <3.0 mmol/L (<116 mg/dL) to <2.0 mmol/L (<77 mg/dL) decreased the risk of vascular disease by about 25%. HPS also provided conclusive evidence of benefit in older patients, over 70 years of age, and in women, who had been excluded from some trials in the past. This trial was also the first to suggest that larger reductions in LDL cholesterol might lead to greater risk reduction.

“Trials suggest that there is no threshold LDL cholesterol below which therapy should not be initiated”

This has subsequently been confirmed in PROVE IT-TIMI 22.[289] This 24-month study in 3745 patients with ACS compared treatment with atorvastatin 80 mg and pravastatin 40 mg and the risk of recurrent MI or cardiac death. It showed that the more intensive lipid-lowering regimen reduced major cardiovascular events by 16%. PROVE IT also looked at the relationship between LDL cholesterol and the inflammatory biomarker CRP. Patients who had high CRP levels (>2.0 mg/L) and LDL cholesterol >1.8 mmol/L (>70 mg/dL) after statin treatment had the highest event rates, whereas those with low CRP levels (<1 mg/L) and LDL cholesterol <1.8 mmol/L (<70 mg/dL) had the lowest rate of recurrent events. This suggests that, although it is important to reduce LDL cholesterol to <1.8 mmol/L, subsequent event-free survival is also linked to reducing inflammation in general and CRP in particular. This notion is supported by results from the REVERSAL study.[290] This study randomly assigned 502 CHD patients to receive “moderate” treatment with pravastatin 40 mg/day or “intensive” treatment with atorvastatin 80 mg/day, using

“In terms of cholesterol lowering it appears that ‘lower is better’ and that patients should be treated to the lowest recommended targets”

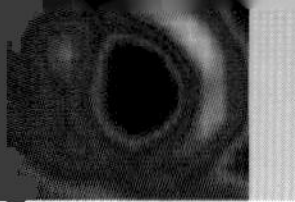

intravascular ultrasound to determine changes in atherosclerosis. This showed that intensive statin treatment reduced the rate of progression of atherosclerosis compared with moderate statin treatment and this was significantly related to greater reductions in the levels of LDL cholesterol and CRP. It would appear therefore that strategies to reduce cardiovascular risk with statins should include monitoring of CRP as well as cholesterol.

"Markers such as CRP may help to identify those who will benefit most from statin treatment"

Data from a meta-analysis of 90,056 patients in 14 randomized trials of statins shows that statins can safely reduce the 5-year incidence of major coronary events, coronary revascularization and stroke by about one fifth per unit mmol/L reduction in LDL cholesterol irrespective of the initial lipid profile.[291]

Data to further consolidate the "lower is better" concept come from the TNT trial.[292] This trial randomized 10,000 CHD patients to assess whether reducing LDL cholesterol beyond 1.9 mmol/L (73 mg/dL) would provide a greater reduction in CHD events than lowering LDL cholesterol more moderately to 2.6 mmol/L (100 mg/dL). Patients with LDL cholesterol <3.4 mmol/L (<131 mg/dL) were randomized to atorvastatin 10 mg/day or atorvastatin 80 mg/day. Patients were followed for a mean of 4.9 years. Results showed that the intensive lipid lowering with atorvastatin 80 mg produced a 22% relative risk reduction in the primary endpoint, although this was associated with a greater incidence of elevated aminotransferase levels. The event rates plotted against LDL cholesterol during statin therapy in the major secondary prevention trials are depicted in Figure 67.[292]

"Agents other than statins can also modify lipid levels, e.g. ezetimibe, fibrates, niacin, fish oils"

The large secondary prevention trials with statins have focused on reducing levels of LDL cholesterol and while reductions in cardiovascular events have been impressive, particularly compared with the

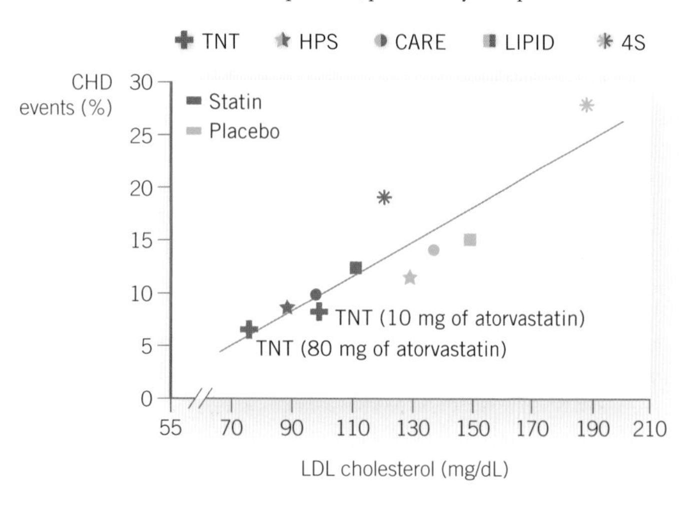

Fig. 67 Event rates plotted against LDL cholesterol levels during statin therapy in secondary prevention studies. Reproduced with permission from La Rosa JC, Grundy SM, Waters DD, et al. Intensive lipid lowering with atorvastatin in patients with coronary artery disease. N Engl J Med 2005;352:1425–1435.

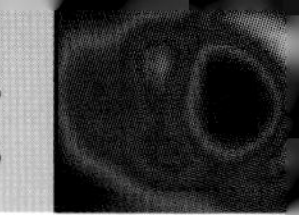

"pre-statin era", significant numbers of events were *not* prevented, as pointed out by Superko.[293] This may be because LDL cholesterol levels were not lowered sufficiently, but it could also signal that poor responders might be explained by the presence of some metabolic abnormality that is not treated solely by LDL reduction. Similarly, monotherapy may be insufficient where multifactorial risk reduction is warranted. European guidelines currently recommend that in patients with clinically established cardiovascular disease and diabetes total plasma cholesterol should be <4.5 mmol/L (<175 mg/dL) and LDL cholesterol <2.5 mmol/L (<100 mg/dL).[294] Forthcoming guidelines are likely to recommend new thresholds for lipid management of total cholesterol <4.0 mmol/L and LDL cholesterol <2.0 mmol/L. Recommendations have been made, based, in part, on review of the above trials, for the US National Cholesterol Education Program Adult Treatment Panel III guidelines to be modified to recommend lower goals and cut-off points for lipid modifying therapy according to categories of risk.[295]

Ezetimibe, a cholesterol absorption inhibitor that prevents cholesterol absorption by inhibiting its passage across the intestinal wall, may also be considered for lipid lowering particularly in patients who are intolerant of statins. It may also be co-administered with a lower dose of statin to improve tolerability.[296] When given as monotherapy ezetimibe lowers LDL cholesterol by 18% and triglycerides by 8%, and increases HDL cholesterol by 1%. When added to a statin ezetimibe provides additional reductions of LDL cholesterol by 25% and triglycerides by 14%, with the additional increase in HDL cholesterol of 3%.[297] Also hsCRP is reduced by an additional 10%. Presently there are no outcome studies with ezetimibe.

"Factors other than LDL cholesterol lowering, such as raising HDL cholesterol or lowering triglycerides may be important in individual patients"

Targets other than LDL cholesterol may need to be addressed in order to achieve event reduction in certain patient groups. Such targets might include HDL cholesterol and apolipoprotein (Apo)-A1, which need to be raised, or triglycerides and levels of Lp(a) and Apo-B, which need to be reduced. Apo-A1 is the major lipoprotein in HDL particles and has a central role in reverse cholesterol transport. Apo-B represents the total number of atherogenic particles. Although Lp(a) is associated with excess cardiovascular risk, there is no evidence yet from clinical trials showing that lowering Lp(a) reduces CHD risk.[298] It is difficult to assess the independent role of triglycerides in CHD risk as the metabolism of both triglycerides and HDL cholesterol are inextricably linked and there is a strong inverse correlation such that increased triglycerides is associated with reduced levels of HDL cholesterol. Statins have only limited effects on triglyceride lowering (-10–14% in the four main secondary prevention trials) and HDL cholesterol raising (+3–8%).

Further candidates in terms of lipid manipulation are HDL cholesterol and its major apolipoprotein Apo-A1, which from observational studies are inversely associated with CHD risk. No prospective trial has been targeted specifically at HDL cholesterol to see whether increasing it can reduce CHD events,[299] in some trials however, particularly with fibrates, a rise in HDL cholesterol seems to contribute to CHD risk reduction.

In terms of currently available therapy other than statins, fibrates are effective in raising HDL and they are beneficial in patients who present with a combination of hypertriglyceridaemia and low HDL cholesterol.[300] Fibrates can stimulate HDL biosynthesis by 6–20% by stimulating hepatic Apo-A1 expression and lipoprotein lipase activity. In VA-HIT[301] CHD patients with HDL cholesterol <40 mg/dL (<1.0 mmol/L) were randomized to gemfibrozil 1200 mg/day or placebo. At 1 year the fibrate-treated patients had increased HDL cholesterol (+6%) and decreased triglycerides (-31%) with no change in LDL cholesterol. At 5 years gemfibrozil decreased non-fatal MI or CHD death by 22% (p=0.001).

> *“Lipid modifying agents other than statins also reduce risk of events in CHD patients”*

A further option is niacin, which raises HDL cholesterol by up to 35% and has been shown to confer a long-term survival benefit in post MI patients.[302] Figure 68 shows the results for cardiovascular endpoints in the Coronary Drug Project (CDP) a randomized trial in 8341 men with previous MI. Of five drug treatment regimens, only niacin significantly reduced risk of events. A more modern, extended-release niacin preparation appears to be better tolerated than older

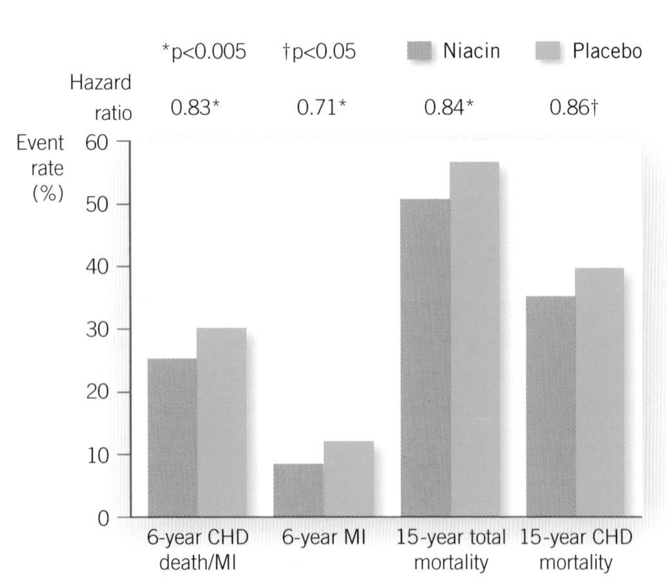

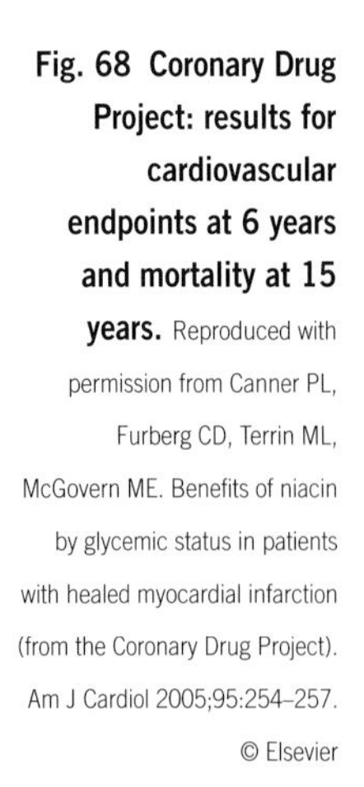
Fig. 68 Coronary Drug Project: results for cardiovascular endpoints at 6 years and mortality at 15 years. Reproduced with permission from Canner PL, Furberg CD, Terrin ML, McGovern ME. Benefits of niacin by glycemic status in patients with healed myocardial infarction (from the Coronary Drug Project). Am J Cardiol 2005;95:254–257. © Elsevier

formulations, which produced a high incidence of side effects, e.g. flushing and other cutaneous reactions.

In terms of secondary prevention another consideration is the use of concentrated fish oil high in omega-3-fatty acids, which reduces high triglyceride levels. One preparation (Omacor) has been shown to reduce sudden cardiac death by 45% when administered as a 1 g capsule daily in survivors of MI.[303]

Hypertension

There is a clear and strong relationship between high blood pressure and CHD. Hypertension contributes to all of the major atherosclerotic cardiovascular disease outcomes, increasing risk, on average, two- to three-fold.[304] Hypertension is also the most consistently powerful predictor of stroke. The risk of recurrent events in patients with CHD is significantly affected by blood pressure levels. Weight reduction can significantly reduce blood pressure and its complications. Treatment with any commonly used blood pressure lowering regimen reduces the risk of total cardiovascular events and larger reductions in blood pressure produce larger reductions in risk.[90] The recently reported ASCOT trial[305] compared the effects on non-fatal MI and fatal CHD among over 19,000 hypertensive patients randomized to atenolol/ bendroflumethiazide or amlodipine/perindopril. The trial was stopped prematurely because the calcium antagonist/ACE inhibitor-based therapy conferred a significant advantage over the beta-blocker/diuretic-based combination on all major cardiovascular endpoints, all-cause mortality and new-onset diabetes. This important finding may influence guidelines and the recommendations on antihypertensive medications and their impact on outcomes in the future. ACE inhibitors have an established role in the treatment of hypertension and LV dysfunction/heart failure. In recent years findings from a number of trials conducted in patients with stable CAD, suggest that ACE inhibitors may also have an important role in preventing cardiovascular events in CAD patients with normal ventricular function.

“High blood pressure increases risk of MI – blood pressure falls with weight reduction”

ACE inhibitors and angiotensin receptor blockers (ARBs)

ACE inhibitors are highly effective in the treatment of hypertension and cardiac failure as well as in the management of acute MI. It has been generally accepted that one of the main mechanisms by which ACE inhibitors produce their beneficial effects is attenuation of the LV dilatation after MI. Evidence from recent clinical studies suggests that other mechanisms, such as anti-atherosclerotic effects or plaque stabilization, may also exist. Similarly, inhibition of the activated renin–angiotensin system has important effects on improving

“One of the main mechansims by which ACE inhibitors produce their beneficial effects is attenuation of the LV dilatation after MI”

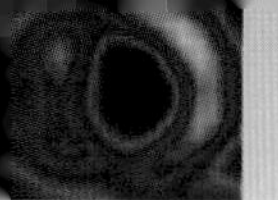

endothelial dysfunction and other properties, which could translate into benefits in all forms of cardiovascular disease including stable CAD.

This view is supported by findings from two major studies, notably the HOPE trial.[306] This was conducted in patients aged 55 years or more at high risk of cardiovascular complications characterized by a high prevalence of diabetes, hypertension, stroke and peripheral vascular disease. HOPE showed a significant 22% reduction in the composite endpoint of MI, stroke, or death from cardiovascular disease among the patients assigned to ramipril. The other major trial was the EUROPA trial[307] conducted in a broader population, all with documented coronary disease without clinical heart failure. The majority were on background therapy of aspirin, statins and beta-blockers. Perindopril treatment was associated with a 20% relative risk reduction in cardiovascular death, MI or cardiac arrest (Figure 69). Importantly there was also a significant 24% reduction in fatal and non-fatal MI. These benefits accrued on top of background treatment with aspirin, beta-blocker and statin and the benefits were independent of these or any other background treatments.

“We cannot assume that ‘all ACE inhibitors are the same’”

These findings are in contrast to the PEACE trial.[308] This trial compared the effects of the ACE inhibitor trandolapril with placebo added to current standard therapy in patients with stable CAD and preserved LV function. The incidence of the primary endpoint – cardiovascular death, MI or coronary revascularization – was almost identical for trandolapril and placebo. The reason why no benefit was demonstrated with the ACE inhibitor is not fully explained. Overall event rates in PEACE were lower than in HOPE or EUROPA and 72% of patients had undergone coronary revascularization. It is also possible that there are inherent differences between individual ACE inhibitors and the doses used, which may in part account for the differential clinical effects seen within studies: we cannot assume that “all ACE inhibitors are the same”.

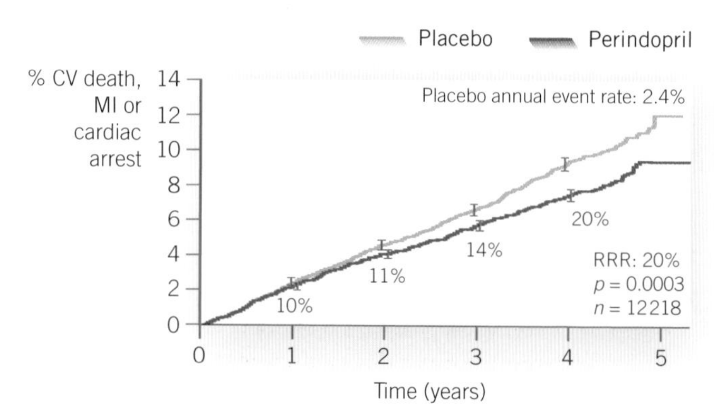

Fig. 69 Results of the EUROPA study. Reproduced with permission from The EUROPA Investigators. Efficacy of perindopril in reduction of cardiovascular events among patients with stable coronary artery disease: randomised, double-blind, placebo-controlled, multicentre trial (the EUROPA study). Lancet 2003;362:782–788. © Elsevier

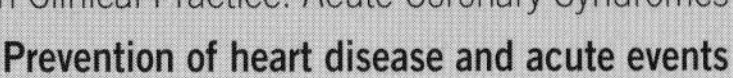

There are insufficient data on ARBs in ACS. The VALIANT trial[309] compared valsartan, captopril, or both in MI complicated by heart failure, LV dysfunction, or both. It showed that valsartan was as effective as captopril in patients who are at high risk of cardiovascular events after MI. Combining these two agents however, increased the incidence of adverse events without improving survival. Further information is awaited on the role of ARBs in CAD patients, presently however trial data support the preferential use of ACE inhibitors in this setting.

Obesity and diabetes

Obesity is literally a growing problem. In the US three out of every 10 adults are obese;[5] rates of obesity in adults and children are also dramatically increasing throughout Europe.[310] Weight reduction may be achieved with physical exercise programmes, which are also associated with favourable metabolic changes including reductions in blood pressure and fasting glucose concentrations, and improvements in the lipid profile. Such changes not only go in the "right direction" in terms of cardiovascular disease prevention, but they may also prevent the development of obesity and/or type 2 diabetes. Several drugs are available for weight reduction. Orlistat, a lipase inhibitor, reduces the absorption of dietary fat and improves lipid and other metabolic parameters. Sibutramine inhibits the reuptake of noradrenaline and serotonin, acting as an appetite suppressant, but is contraindicated in some cardiovascular conditions. A new investigational agent, rimonabant, which selectively blocks the endocannabinoid system (which plays a role in food intake and energy expenditure), has been shown to promote weight loss and also improve lipids and other metabolic parameters (Figure 70).[311] There are currently no outcome studies with these agents.

"Excess weight increases risk of diabetes and most diabetic patients die of cardiovascular causes"

Diabetes increases cardiovascular mortality four- to six-fold and CHD mortality two- to four-fold. Patients who develop this condition have a worse survival prognosis than patients with CHD who do not have diabetes. About 80% of diabetic patients will die of cardiovascular causes. Aggressive control of blood pressure appears to be key in reducing macrovascular events in diabetes. Preliminary reports suggest that glitazones such as pioglitazone and rosiglitazone exert favourable effects on lipids in diabetic patients. The PROACTIVE study is a European investigation of the effects of pioglitazone on morbidity and mortality associated with cardiovascular disease progression in over 5000 patients with type 2 diabetes. Preliminary findings[312] showed no significant difference between pioglitazone and placebo in the composite endpoint of fatal and non-fatal cardiovascular events. However further analysis revealed that pioglitazone was associated with a significant reduction in risk of death, stroke or MI, but it was

"About 80% of diabetic patients will die of cardiovascular causes"

Fig. 70 Change in HDL cholesterol and triglycerides. One-year results of the RIO-Europe trial.[311]

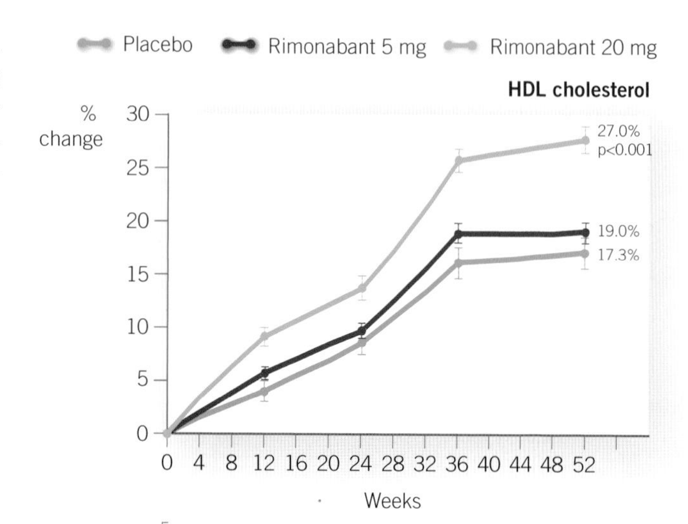

ITT LOCF
- Placebo : 13.4%
- 5 mg : 16.2 % (p=0.048 versus placebo)
- 20 mg : 22.3 % (p<0.001 versus placebo)

“Rimonabant has been shown to promote weight loss and also improve lipids and other metabolic parameters”

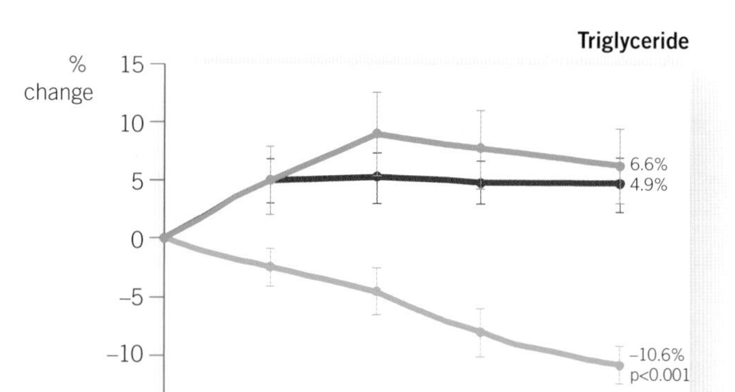

ITT LOCF
- Placebo : 8.3 %
- 5 mg : 5.7 % (not significant versus placebo)
- 20 mg : –6.8 % (p<0.001 versus placebo)

also associated with a 1.6% increase in heart failure admissions. The analysis of these results has been strongly criticized,[313] as, in the absence of significance in the primary endpoint, analysis of secondary endpoints has little value. However the glitazones may still have demonstrable cardiovascular benefits, which may be confirmed in future studies.

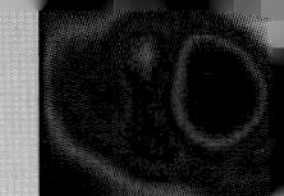

Exercise training

Exercise training, as well as its role in CHD prevention, is also integral to any cardiac rehabilitation programme, and it has been shown to slow the progression of, or partially reduce, the severity of coronary atherosclerosis. Such programmes are also associated with lower total and cardiac mortality rates compared with usual medical care.[314] It has also been suggested however that standard cardiac rehabilitation is less effective for diabetic patients and it may be that diabetic patients warrant specialized programmes of rehabilitation to integrate the care of their condition with their recent MI.

“Exercise training, as well as its role in CHD prevention, is also integral to any cardiac rehabilitation programme”

Conclusions

It has been calculated that about two-thirds to three-quarters of future vascular events could be prevented in high-risk patients by the use of aspirin, beta-blocker, statin and ACE inhibitor (Figure 71).[315] These drugs reduce the risk of future vascular events by about 25% each and the benefits of each intervention appear to be largely independent. Additionally there is the potential to lower risk by about one-half by quitting smoking and about one-quarter by reducing systolic blood pressure by 10 mmHg.

Similar calculations have been made by Wald and Law.[316] They suggest that more than 80% of cardiovascular events could be reduced if everyone over the age of 55 years and all patients with vascular disease were to take a “Polypill” comprising a dose of statin, thiazide diuretic, beta-blocker, ACE inhibitor, folic acid and aspirin. This hypothesis has not been tested.

This short review has looked at some of the major cardiovascular risk factors and their management. Space precludes us looking at other important factors including, for example, psychological stress. Depression is common following an episode of UA and is associated

“There is no excuse for not implementing programmes for prevention in those who are at risk of or who already have manifest disease”

	Relative risk reduction	2-year event rate
None	-	8%
Aspirin	25%	6%
Beta-blockers	25%	4.5%
Lipid-lowering (by 1.5 mmol/L; 58 mg/dL)	30%	3%
ACE inhibitors	25%	2.3%
Cumulative relative risk reduction if all four drugs used is about 75%		

Fig. 71 Potential cumulative impact of four secondary preventive treatments. Reproduced with permission from Yusuf S. Two decades of progress in preventing vascular disease. Lancet 2002;360:2–3. © Elsevier

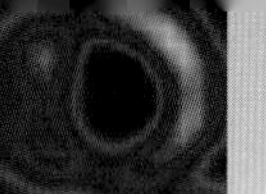

with an increased risk of major cardiac events during the following year.[317]

Both primary and secondary prevention of CHD are major public health issues. There is ample evidence that intervention reduces risk of development of events and risk of reinfarction in patients with established CHD. There is no excuse for not implementing programmes for prevention in those who are at risk of or who already have manifest disease.

“Inflammation plays a key role in atherosclerosis and its clinical sequelae”

Antibiotic therapy

Recent evidence suggests that atherosclerosis – once deemed a degenerative disease – is an active inflammatory and thrombotic disease.[21] It has been proposed that micro-organisms may trigger the inflammation and hence the atherosclerotic process. The “infective”

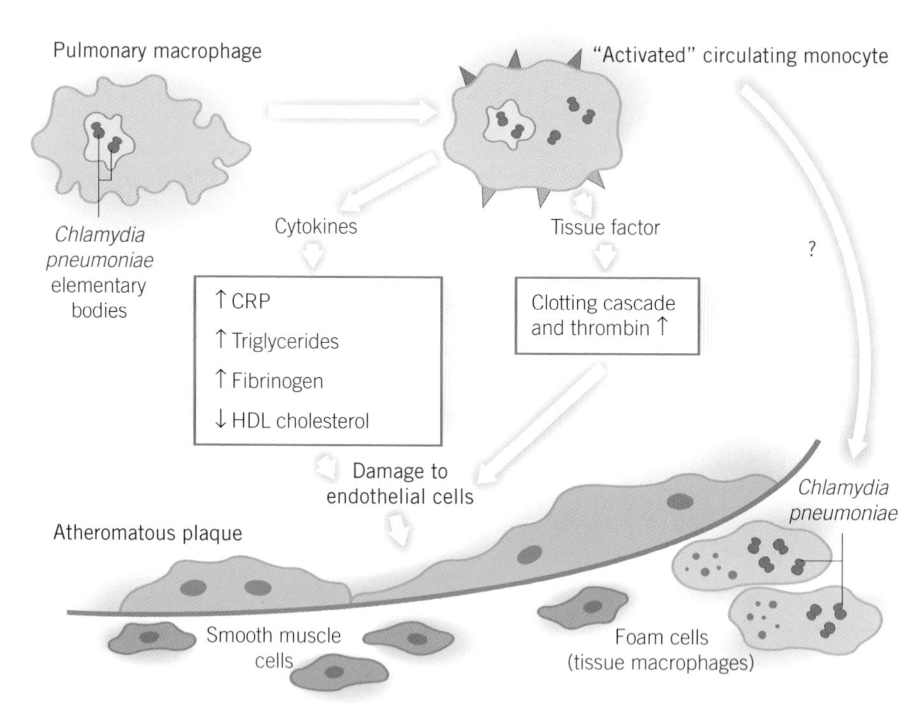

Fig. 72 Possible mechanisms for the involvement of *C. pneumoniae* in atherogenesis. Infection with *C. pneumoniae* may induce a chronic immune activation, mediated by cytokines, that contributes to direct endothelial cell damage or stimulates the synthesis of acute phase reactants such as fibrinogen and CRP. In parallel, chronic infection may also increase expression of monocyte derived procoagulants such as tissue factor and thereby increase the risk of local or distant thrombosis.

Reproduced from Gupta S, Camm AJ. Chlamydia pneumoniae and coronary heart disease. BMJ 1997;314:1778–1779.

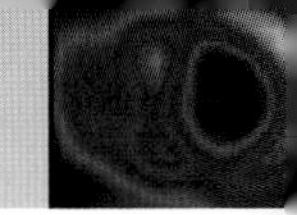

hypothesis – first proposed more than a century ago by Virchow – has been recently pursued with vigour. The greatest body of evidence suggests *Chlamydia pneumoniae*, a common respiratory pathogen, is the main "culprit" microorganism.[318] Consistent findings of bacterial antigens, DNA and occasionally live "viable" organisms within the human atherosclerotic plaque support *C. pneumoniae*'s link with atherogenesis.[319,320] In addition, animal models have shown how atherosclerosis may be induced by endovascular infection with *C. pneumoniae*;[321] and *in vitro* studies have explored various immunological and inflammatory pathways linking infection and atherothrombosis (Figure 72). Antibiotic trials have been performed to assess whether there is any role for anti-chlamydial agents in the prevention of cardiovascular events.

"Several lines of evidence have implicated chronic infection (in particular with C. pneumoniae*) in atherosclerosis"*

Early antibiotic studies in CHD

The first two independent pilot studies exploring antibiotics in patients with CHD were published in 1997. Both these studies demonstrated that short courses of macrolide antibiotics produced a reduction in cardiovascular events compared with placebo.[322,323] However longer-term follow-up suggested effects were not sustained beyond 18 months.

The ACADEMIC, STAMINA, ANTIBIO and ISAR-3 studies reported mixed findings.[324–327] STAMINA showed a 36% reduction in major events in those receiving antibiotic-containing regimens compared with placebo (p=0.02), independent of confounding factors, while ISAR-3 showed that PCI patients with high levels of antibodies to *C. pneumoniae* benefited from a month of roxithromycin in terms of less restenosis and fewer revascularization procedures. In contrast both ACADEMIC and ANTIBIO showed no clinical benefit, however it was not totally negative. In ACADEMIC there were changes in certain systemic markers of inflammation (CRP, TNF-alpha, and Il-1 and Il-6) following 3 months' azithromycin, and low recruitment and poor compliance with therapy in ANTIBIO were thought, in part, to explain the negative findings.

"Preliminary pilot studies suggested that antibiotic treatment may reduce the risk of further cardiovascular events; this has been refuted by larger randomized trials"

The results of preliminary antibiotic studies (Figure 73) were encouraging and left open the potential for a modest-to-moderate antibiotic benefit in CHD and ACS. However some of the above-mentioned studies were limited by small sample size, lack of adequate statistical power and arbitrary duration of antibiotic therapy.

Antibiotics in non-coronary vascular disease

Antibiotic trials utilizing non-invasive measurements of abdominal aortic aneurysm (AAA) growth, carotid artery thickness and peripheral

Fig. 73 Early antibiotic studies for prevention of cardiovascular events.

Trial (year)	Study population	Antibiotic	Results
London study (1997)	Post MI n=220	Azithromycin 3–6 days	Positive
ROXIS (1997)	ACS n=202	Roxithromycin 30 days	Positive at 1 month Negative at 3 and 6 months
Washington study (1998)	Post PCI n=88	Azithromycin 28 days	Positive
ACADEMIC (1999)	Stable CHD n=302	Azithromycin 3 months	Negative
Bangkok study (2001)	ACS n=84	Roxithromycin 30 days	Negative
STAMINA (2002)	ACS n=325	Azithromycin or amoxicillin and metronidazole 7 days	Positive
CLARIFY (2002)	ACS n=148	Clarithromycin 3 months	Positive

vascular disease symptoms have shown encouraging results (Figure 74).[328,329] Although these studies showed a positive effect of the antibiotic on regression of atherosclerosis in arterial vasculature, more recent data suggest only a temporary benefit.[330]

Large randomized control trials with antibiotics (Figure 75)

WIZARD was the first large randomized trial.[331] Over 7000 stable patients with a history of MI and seropositivity to *C. pneumoniae* were

Fig. 74 Antibiotic trials in non-coronary vascular disease.

Investigators	Population	N	Antibiotic	Course	Follow-up	Results
Mosorin *et al*	AAA growth	32	Doxycycline	3 months	18 months	Positive, $p<0.05$
Vammen *et al*	AAA growth	92	Roxithromycin	28 days	18 months	Positive, $p=0.02$
Wiesli *et al*	Peripheral vascular disease	40	Roxithromycin	28 days	30 months	Positive, $p<0.05$
Sander *et al*	Carotid thickness	272	Roxithromycin	30 days	24 months	Positive, $p<0.01$
Sander *et al*	Restenosis	1010	Roxithromycin	28 days	12 months	-/+

-/+ indicates negative overall but positive in subjects with *C. pneumoniae* antibody titre >512

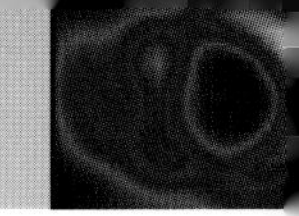

randomized to receive either placebo or 3 months of azithromycin (600 mg/week). Overall, short-term (3-month) azithromycin therapy was safe and well tolerated. However it resulted in only a 7% reduction in the incidence of the primary endpoint (composite of death, MI, hospitalization for UA, and need for revascularization). No evidence of a treatment effect by baseline *C. pneumoniae* titre was observed. However *post hoc* analyses suggested a possible benefit during and shortly after treatment (33% reduction in death or MI at 6 months, p=0.03), which was not sustained over the observation period, but also greater benefit with other risk factors such as diabetes mellitus and hyperlipidaemia (unpublished data). This raised the question of whether more prolonged antimicrobial therapy (in a targeted group) may have produced clinical benefit. In contrast the ACES study with the longest antibiotic regimen of over 12 months in 4000 adults with stable CHD randomized to oral azithromycin 600 mg once a week or placebo showed no difference between the groups for composite cardiovascular endpoints.[332]

“Issues such as optimal antibiotic regimens, duration of therapy, relevance of other infections (including viruses) and concomitant secondary prevention medication suggest further research and studies could be considered”

The AZACS study examined approximately 1450 patients in acute cardiac settings.[333] Patients were entered regardless of whether serology to *C. pneumoniae* was positive or negative. Treatment was given with azithromycin for only 5 days and duration of follow-up was 6 months. No benefit upon ischaemic endpoints was observed. The AZACS study indicated with reasonable power and reliability that there is no important benefit of this short treatment regimen of azithromycin beginning at the time of ACS.[333]

Finally PROVE-IT randomized 3000 patients with ACS in a 2 x 2 factorial design. Treatments included:

Fig. 75 Prospective randomized control antibiotic trials for CHD prevention.

Trial	Population	N	Antibiotic	Course	Follow-up	Results
WIZARD	Stable CHD	7724	Azithromycin	3 months	3 years	Non-significant
AZACS	ACS	1439	Azithromycin	5 days	6 months	Non-significant
ANTIBIO	ACS	872	Roxithromycin	6 weeks	1 year	Negative
ACES	Stable CHD	4000	Azithromycin	Weekly for 1 year	4 years	Non-significant
PROVE-IT	ACS	4000+	Gatifloxacin	2 weeks, 10 days	Monthly for 2 years	Negative
ISAR-3	PCI	1000+	Roxithromycin	1 month	6–12 months	Probably positive
ANTIBIOS	Post-MI	872	Roxithromycin	6 weeks		Negative

1. One of the two statin regimens (pravastatin or atorvastatin).
2. An intermittent course of the quinolone gatifloxacin or placebo.

It was hypothesized that quinolone therapy offered potentially superior bactericidal activity against *C. pneumoniae.* Unfortunately no differences were noted between the groups given antibiotics or no antibiotics with regard to major cardiovascular events.[334]

Conclusion

"There is no current role for antibiotics in the management of CHD; the focus remains on controlling the conventional risk factors"

The early favourable results from preliminary antibiotic studies have not translated into similar findings with the larger trials. The ongoing debate includes:

- Issues of choice of antibiotics (bacteriostatic versus bacteriocidal).
- Whether combination antimicrobial regimens would be required (analogous to the treatment of tuberculosis).
- Whether the co-administration of steroids (to ensure that the organism is replicating or viable and hence more sensitive to antibiotics) would be worth pursuing.

It is acknowledged that perhaps targeted therapy may have shown more favourable findings rather than selecting a wide range of cardiac patients with multiple risk factors and varied antibody levels to *C. pneumoniae.* In addition the duration of therapy, now tested up to 1 year (ACES study), has been another contention and up until now has been relatively arbitrary in study design.

Infection may be associated with atherosclerosis and its clinical sequelae. However recent randomized trials have failed to show the clinical benefits of antibiotics in subjects with CHD.[335–338] Indeed, a recent meta-analysis of clinical trials of anti-chlamydial antibiotic therapy in patients with CAD (11 reports, 19,217 patients) concluded that currently available evidence does not demonstrate an overall benefit of antibiotic therapy in reducing mortality or cardiovascular events.[339] While the infection hypothesis may merit continued exploration, at this juncture our focus remains on treating and addressing traditional risk factors for CHD with no role for antibiotics in the treatment of CHD. We are alerted to the landmark INTERHEART study (covering data from 52 countries), which reminds us that 90% of MIs worldwide are explained by five main risk factors – hypertension, diabetes mellitus, cigarette smoking, abnormal lipid profile and lack of physical activity.[276] This is where our efforts should currently lie and the hypothesis of "infection and atherosclerosis" remain an intriguing research issue.

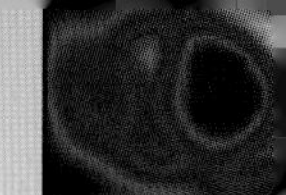

Case study 1

Atypical chest pain

Mrs HE, a 64-year-old female widow, presented to the GP surgery complaining of 1-month left-sided chest pain. The discomfort was intermittent, occurring both at rest and with physical effort and lasting 5 to 15 minutes. Symptoms had been increasing in frequency with four to five episodes in the past week. On the day of presentation she noted slight shortness of breath. Her GP obtained an ECG which showed non-specific T wave inversion in the lateral leads (Figure 76). No old ECG was available for comparison.

In the office the patient described persistent left-sided chest discomfort with heaviness in the left shoulder. CAD risk factors were "negative" for smoking, hypertension, and diabetes mellitus. Family history included a mother with a history of ischaemic heart disease (IHD) at age 62. Past medical history included oesophagitis. Medications: none.

“The patient described persistent left-sided chest discomfort with heaviness in the left shoulder”

Investigation	Result
Total cholesterol	5.4 mmol/L
HDL cholesterol	1.51 mmol/L
LDL cholesterol	3.21 mmol/L
Total:HDL ratio	3.6

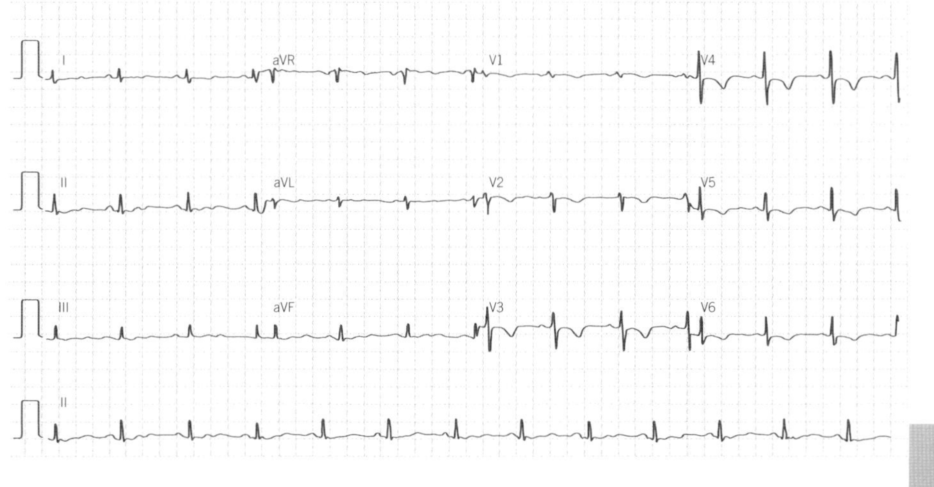

Fig. 76 ECG showing non-specific T wave inversion in the lateral leads.

"Final diagnosis was noncardiac chest pain most likely musculoskeletal in origin"

Comment and management

She was immediately referred to the casualty department where she received sublingual glyceryl trinitrate without relief. Aspirin, a statin and metoprolol were initiated and the pain subsided spontaneously over 2 hours. Serial ECGs were unchanged and troponins x3 were in the normal range. A stress echocardiogram was performed but the patient only exercised 4.5 metabolic equivalents (METS) stopping due to fatigue and mild chest discomfort. The monitored ECG developed 1 mV horizontal ST depression but the echo images showed normal resting left ventricular function with normal enhanced contractility of all wall segments. Due to the submaximal exercise effort a cardiac catheterization was obtained revealing mild luminal irregularity with plaque disease no tighter than 25% luminal diameter.

Final diagnosis was noncardiac chest pain most likely musculoskeletal in origin. Symptoms abated after empiric treatment with nonsteroidal anti-inflammatory medication. Secondary prevention for IHD was continued.

- **Prolonged chest pain at rest without dynamic ECG changes and negative cardiac biomarkers is unlikely to represent ACS**
- **A regular treadmill exercise test has low specificity when there are ST-T wave abnormalities on the resting ECG. A stress test with imaging (either stress echocardiogram or stress nuclear study) is preferred**
- **A treadmill stress test with submaximal effort has low sensitivity for detecting CAD. Alternatives to improve diagnostic accuracy include a pharmacologic stress imaging study (either dobutamine stress echo or persantin/adenosine nuclear study) or diagnostic catheterization**

Case study 2

Recurrent MI in elderly woman

"Patient had a history of MI"

Mrs DC is an 87-year-old lady with new onset persistent chest pain. The patient had a history of MI in 1988 but no further cardiac symptoms. Recently she had a hip fracture requiring insertion of a hip screw and follow-up physiotherapy without cardiac complications. On the morning of admission there was onset of moderate chest pain accompanied by shortness of breath. Symptoms continued for 1.5 hours despite two puffs of glyceryl trinitrate sublingual spray.

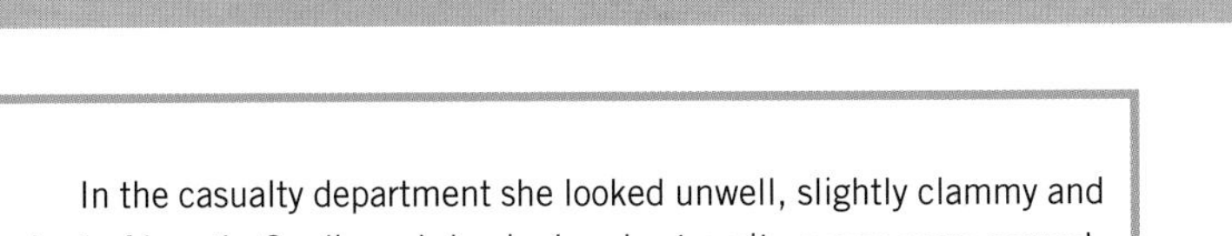

In the casualty department she looked unwell, slightly clammy and short of breath. Cardiac, abdominal and extremity exams were normal. An ECG during pain showed diffuse ST depression in leads I, II, L, F, V4-6 (Figure 77). Aspirin 300 mg, frusemide 40 mg and intravenous heparin were started and the patient was admitted to hospital.

Investigation	Result
Pulse rate	80 beats/minute
Blood pressure	150/80 mmHg
Chest examination	Bibasal crepitations and slight wheezes
ECG	Diffuse ST depression
Troponin	Positive

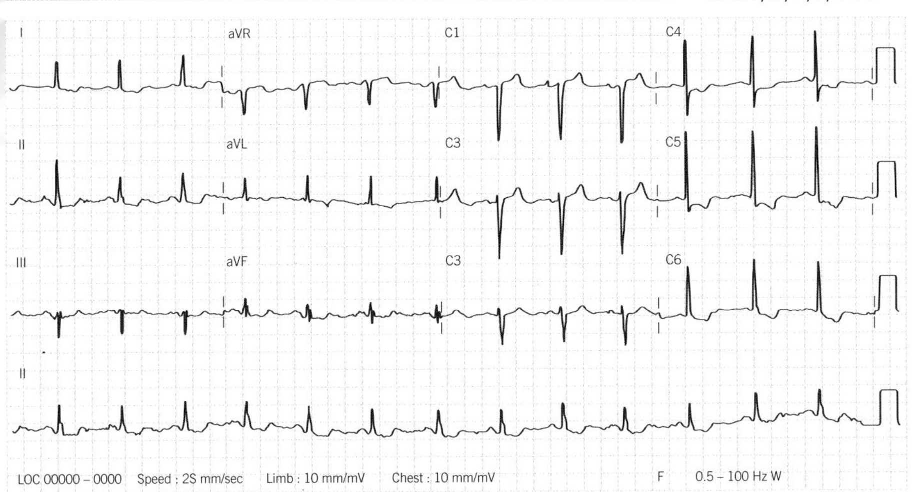

Fig. 77 ECG showing diffuse ST depression in leads I, II, L, F, V4-6.

Comment and management

She was treated for NSTEMI with clopidogrel and propranolol. An echocardiogram demonstrated lateral wall hypokinesis with an ejection fraction of 45%. All symptoms subsided within 24 hours of initiation of therapy. Follow-up ECG showed partial improvement of the ST depression. Transfer to a hospital with catheterization facilities was considered but conservative medical treatment was continued due to the patient's age. Additional secondary prevention medications were started including a statin and an ACE inhibitor. The patient remained asymptomatic and was discharged on her medical regimen.

“Transfer to a hospital with catheterization facilities was considered”

"Medical therapy for NSTEMI should include dual antiplatelet therapy"

- **Thrombolytic therapy is not used to treat NSTEMI**
- **In the elderly the decision to treat conservatively or with PCI should be based on clinical and social factors. PCI can be performed successfully in the elderly but this is often chosen when the patient cannot be stabilized medically**
- **Medical therapy for NSTEMI should include dual antiplatelet therapy (aspirin and clopidogrel)**

Case study 3

Unstable angina in an elderly man

Mr MF is an 84-year-old male retired shopkeeper brought to Casualty by ambulance complaining of left-sided chest pain. Symptoms started the night before and were intermittent up until hospitalization. In Casualty he received buccal glyceryl trinitrate with partial relief. Medical history was negative for IHD. Coronary risk factors were negative for hypertension, hyperlipidaemia, diabetes, and family history of CAD. He smoked heavily in the past but stopped 5 years ago. Past medical history included mild COPD.

"Medical history was negative for ischaemic heart disease"

Investigation	Result
Blood pressure	138/78 mmHg
Heart rate	100 beats/minute (regular)
Chest examination	"Dry" crackles on inspiration, otherwise normal
Chest X-ray	Unremarkable
ECG	Sinus rhythm with T wave inversion in leads II, III, aVF
Troponin I	Negative

Comment and management

The patient was admitted and started on aspirin, LMWH, metoprolol, and clopidogrel. Symptoms did not recur and serial cardiac biomarkers remained normal. After discussion with the patient it was decided to continue conservative medical therapy rather than invasive treatment pending results of an exercise treadmill test.

"Serial cardiac biomarkers remained normal"

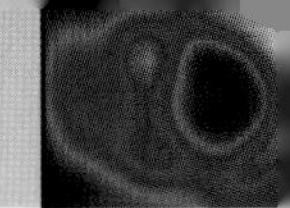

- **Intermittent pain over several hours warrants observation in hospital**
- **Baseline ECG and cardiac biomarkers (troponin) are mandatory initial tests immediately upon arrival at a medical facility. These tests will categorize the patient as having either UA or NSTEMI**
- **Current treatment of UA includes aspirin, beta-blockers, heparin (unfractionated or low molecular weight) and, in most cases, a thienopyridine (clopidogrel)**
- **A GP IIb/IIIa inhibitor is not needed if troponins are negative and there are no plans for urgent catheterization**
- **Conservative medical versus invasive therapy should be based on patient age, response to medical therapy, associated medical conditions and performance on exercise treadmill testing**
- **Discharge medication should include aspirin, beta-blockers and statins indefinitely, if tolerated. Clopidogrel should be continued for at least 9 months. ACE inhibitors may also be considered indefinitely**

"Baseline ECG and cardiac biomarkers are mandatory initial tests"

Case study 4

Transfer for PCI

Mr GW, a 57-year-old ship-builder, was admitted to a District General Hospital with a 90-minute history of central chest pain beginning while at work. He had no prior cardiac history. CAD risk factors were limited to a 30 packet year history of smoking.

Admission vital signs were blood pressure 145/78 mmHg, heart rate 98 beats per minute. Initial ECG showed 4 mV ST elevation in leads V1–5. Thrombolytic therapy was instituted immediately in the casualty unit (door-to-needle time 20 minutes). Other medical treatment included beta-blocker, aspirin, statin, ACE inhibitor, and a 48-hour infusion of UFH.

"Initial ECG showed 4 mV ST elevation"

Chest pain nearly disappeared and ST segments partially resolved within 30 minutes of infusion. Two and half hours later however, severe chest pain recurred with 8 mV ST elevation in the anterior leads. Emergency transfer to a hospital with PCI and surgical backup was activated. Prior to transfer the patient was loaded with clopidogrel 600 mg.

Comment and management

Cardiac catheterization was performed immediately upon arrival at the receiving hospital. Angiography revealed normal left main, subtotal obstruction of the proximal LAD artery (TIMI 1 flow), 70% narrowing of the dominant left circumflex, and a normal small right coronary artery

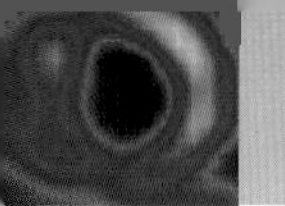

“There was a severe discrete stenosis in the mid-LAD coronary artery”

(RCA). A drug-eluting stent was placed in the LAD with restoration of TIMI 3 flow (Figure 78).

Peak CK was 177 iu/L and troponin I was 4.86 μg/L. Echocardiogram revealed mild anterior hypokinesis with an ejection fraction of 48%. The patient was discharged 3 days later on aspirin, clopidogrel, beta-blocker, ACE inhibitor, and a statin.

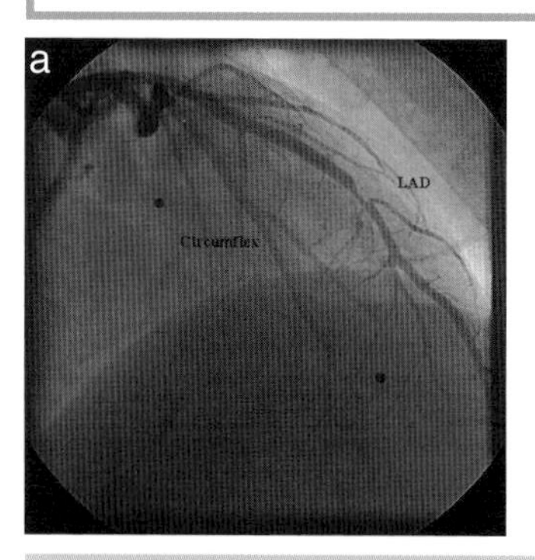

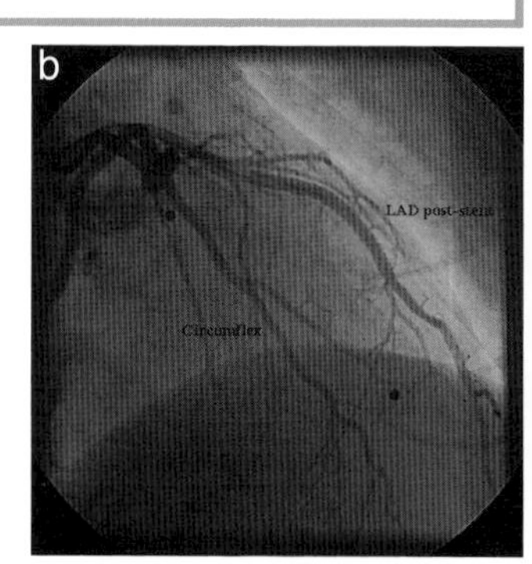

Fig. 78 Coronary angiographs: a. pre-PCI showing obstructed LAD coronary artery; b. post-PCI showing TIMI 3 flow down LAD.

- **All chest pain patients should get an ECG immediately upon arrival at the casualty unit**
- **For patients with STEMI door-to-needle time for administration of thrombolytic drug should be less than 30 minutes**
- **A GP IIb/IIIa inhibitor is usually administered in conjunction with stent placement, but this drug is contraindicated in patients who have received full-dose thrombolytic therapy**
- **An ACE inhibitor should be added to the secondary prevention regimen post anterior MI even when the ejection fraction is preserved**

Case study 5

Crescendo angina

“Two-week history of new-onset exertional chest pain culminating in chest discomfort at rest”

Mr GD, a 68-year-old man, was admitted to an outlying hospital with a 2-week history of new-onset exertional chest pain culminating in chest discomfort at rest for 1 hour. Upon arrival at the hospital he had mild residual chest pain. There was no prior history of CAD. Coronary risk factors included hyperlipidaemia (fasting total cholesterol 6.9 mmol/L prior to treatment), and hypertension. Family history was negative. He had smoked for 5 years but stopped over 25 years ago, and there was no diabetes. Past medical history comprised Dukes C carcinoma of the

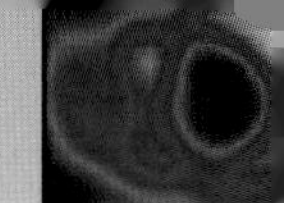

Medications	**Low-dose aspirin**
	Statin
	ACE inhibitor
Blood pressure	**118/76 mmHg**
Heart rate	**78 beats/minute**
Physical exam	**Normal**

colon 5 years ago treated with hemicolectomy and 6 months' adjuvant chemotherapy.

Admission ECG showed anterolateral T wave inversion and troponin I was normal (<0.15 μg/L). Initial treatment included aspirin, iv glyceryl trinitrate, beta-blocker, subcutaneous LMWH, and iv GP IIb/IIIa inhibitor. Chest pain resolved after 2 hours' treatment but the second troponin I increased to 0.40 μg/L suggestive of a NSTEMI. At that time the patient was transferred to a hospital with interventional cardiac catheterization capability with surgical backup. Upon transfer the patient developed recurrent moderate chest pain with 2 mV ST depression in V1–V4.

Comment and management

The patient was brought to the catherization laboratory and an intra-aortic balloon was inserted with resolution of chest discomfort. Left ventriculography demonstrated minor anterior hypokinesia. Coronary arteriography showed a normal left main, a 95% proximal LAD stenosis with intraluminal clot, left circumflex luminal irregularity, and a 90% mid-vessel RCA stenosis. Drug-eluting stents were placed in the LAD and RCA with TIMI 3 flow and no complications (Figure 79).

The GP IIb/IIIa inhibitor was continued for 12 hours and the IABP removed the next day. Peak CK was 227 iu/L and troponin I was 2.85 μg/L. He was discharged well 3 days after his admission.

“An intra-aortic balloon was inserted with resolution of chest discomfort”

“This patient was high-risk ACS with TIMI risk score 5”

- **This patient was high-risk ACS with TIMI risk score 5 (chest pain within past 48 hours, ECG changes, positive biomarkers, >2 CAD risk factors, on aspirin)**
- **A GP IIb/IIIa inhibitor should be added to the treatment of ACS when the troponin is “positive” and PCI is planned**
- **Patients at high risk who might benefit from revascularization should be transferred to a facility with PCI and surgical capability**
- **IABP can be helpful to stabilize a patient with medically refractory ischaemia**

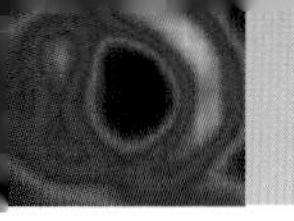

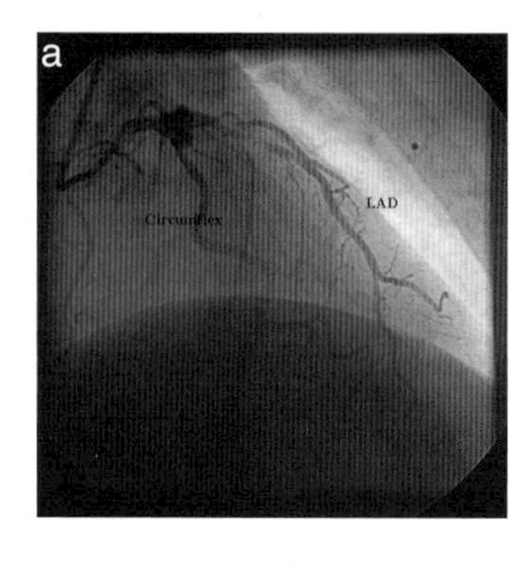

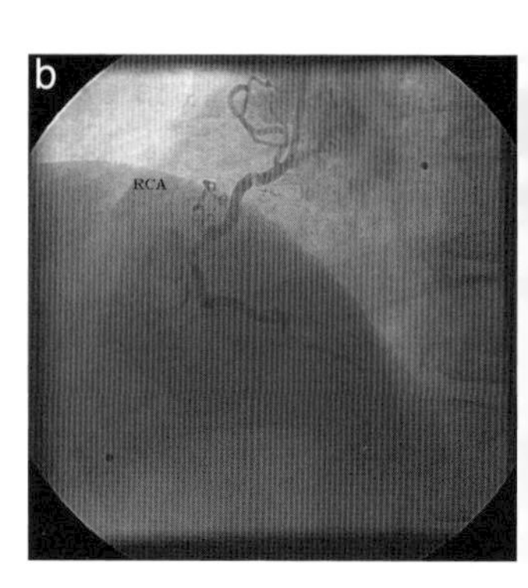

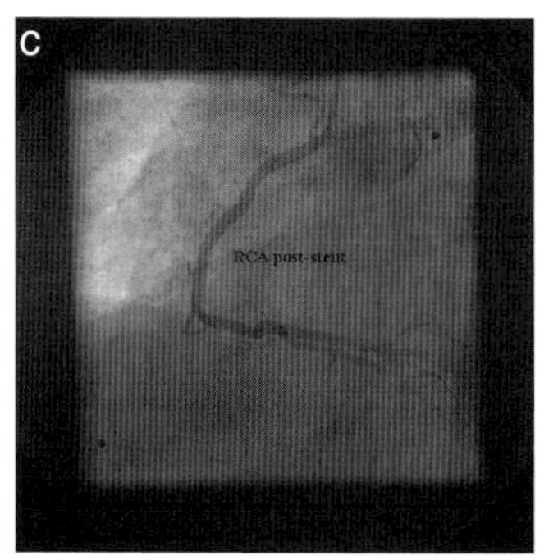

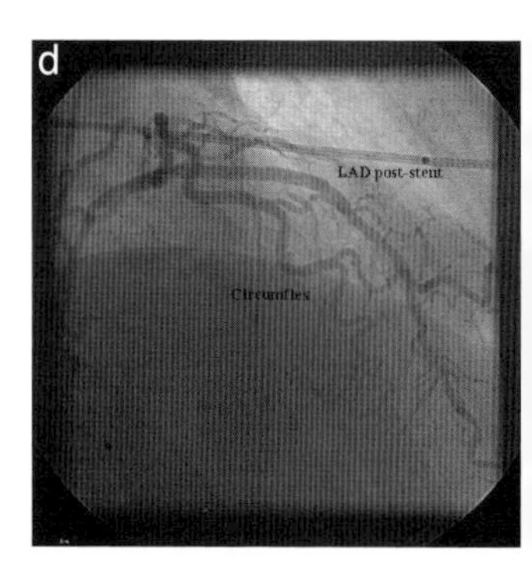

Fig. 79 Coronary angiographs: a. pre-PCI showing non-dominant circumflex artery with diffuse mild atheroma only; b. pre-PCI showing 90% stenosis in mid-vessel dominant RCA; c. peri-PCI – a second drug-eluting stent is inserted overlapping and proximal to the first; d. post-PCI a further drug-eluting stent is inserted into the LAD.

Case study 6

Progressive coronary artery disease

Mrs KE is a 65-year-old woman with early-onset CAD. At age 50 she presented with atypical chest pain. Cardiac risk factors included hypertension, mild hyperlipidaemia and obesity. An exercise treadmill test was nondiagnostic due to submaximal exercise effort limited by dyspnoea. An upper endoscopy demonstrated mild oesophagitis and the patient was treated with H_2 blockers with good response. Other medications included atenolol 25 mg/day, simvastatin 10 mg/day and aspirin.

Ten months later the patient had recurrent chest pain particularly associated with an exertion. An adenosine stress nuclear perfusion test was obtained revealing lateral ischaemia. Medical therapy was adjusted to include atenolol 50 mg/day and diltiazem 30 mg three times daily. Despite these medications, chest pain recurred and the patient underwent cardiac catheterization. Coronary angiography demonstrated

“An adenosine stress nuclear perfusion test was obtained revealing lateral ischaemia”

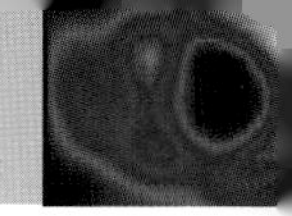

normal left main, mild narrowing of the RCA, minimal irregularity of the LAD vessel, and severe 85–90% narrowing of a small lateral circumflex branch. Medical therapy was readjusted increasing diltiazem to 60 mg three times daily.

Six months later the patient suffered an inferior wall MI. Repeat catheterization showed new 100% obstruction of the RCA. A bare metal stent was positioned in the RCA with restoration of antegrade flow. The patient was discharged on aspirin and ticlopidine 250 mg twice daily but after 2 days she stopped the ticlopidine due to gastrointestinal distress. Six days later she was readmitted with chest pain and inferior ST elevation on ECG. Catheterization demonstrated acute thrombosis of the RCA stent, which was recanalized with balloon angioplasty. The patient was discharged 4 days later on clopidogrel 75 mg once daily and remains asymptomatic.

“Catheterization demonstrated acute thrombosis of the RCA stent”

- **Patients unable to perform a treadmill exercise test should be considered for a pharmacologic stress nuclear study or stress echocardiogram**
- **Dual antiplatelet therapy with aspirin and a thienopyridine (ticlopidine or clopidogrel) is needed to minimize risk of early acute stent thrombosis**
- **Acute MI often results from plaque rupture and thrombosis of vessels with non-critical coronary stenoses**
- **Progression of CAD with plaque stabilization and possibly regression can be prevented by high-dose statin therapy**

Case study 7

STEMI

Mrs SC, a 60-year-old woman, was admitted to a District General Hospital with a 2.5 hour history of chest pain that had begun while playing badminton. She had a 30 packet year history of cigarette smoking but no other cardiac risk factors. She had no previous cardiac history.

Her admission ECG showed 4 mV ST elevation in the inferior leads with ST depression in V1–3. Soon after arrival in the Accident and Emergency department the patient suffered a cardiac arrest. She received 20 minutes of cardio-pulmonary resuscitation (CPR) including a total of 13 DC shocks for ventricular fibrillation. She was intubated and ventilated. Once a cardiac output was restored the patient was extubated and half-dose iv thrombolytic agent was administered. There was no apparent neurologic deficit. Ninety minutes post thrombolysis,

“Half-dose intravenous thrombolytic agent was administered”

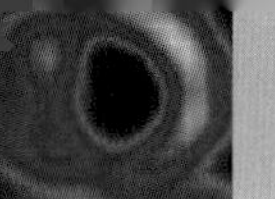

the ST segment elevation had failed to resolve. She was therefore transferred emergently to a Regional Hospital for catheterization and possible rescue PCI.

Comment and management

"On arrival the patient was in cardiogenic shock"

On arrival the patient was in cardiogenic shock with a systolic blood pressure of 65 mmHg and oliguria. Coronary angiography revealed a normal left main coronary, 100% chronic LAD occlusion with bridging collaterals, and mild left circumflex irregularity. The RCA had proximal subtotal occlusion with visible thrombus and TIMI 1 flow. An abciximab bolus was administered and a drug eluting stent positioned at the site of RCA stenosis. TIMI 3 flow was achieved and blood pressure rose to 95 mmHg with return of urination. Her CK peaked at 7848 iu/L with a troponin I of >50 µg/L. Over the next day the patient stabilized in the cardiac high dependency unit and was transferred to the telemetry floor. Echocardiography demonstrated inferoposterior akinesis with an estimated ejection fraction of 48%. Medications were adjusted including aspirin, clopidogrel, a beta-blocker, a statin and an ACE inhibitor. The patient was discharged 7 days after admission.

"Prolonged CPR (>10 minutes) is considered a relative contraindication for fibrinolysis"

- **Early thrombolytic therapy is beneficial especially when administered in the first 3 hours of onset of chest pain. In this patient however, prolonged CPR (>10 minutes) is considered a relative contraindication for fibrinolysis. The decision to use a thrombolytic agent should be based on the availability of rapid transfer to a hospital with interventional catheterization capability and other clinical factors (e.g. electrical stability, rib trauma from the CPR)**
- **Half-dose thrombolytic has been used to reduce risk of bleeding when there is the likely need to give a GP IIb/IIIa inhibitor in conjunction with emergency PCI. The safety and efficacy of this combination treatment is not fully established**
- **Failure to resolve ST elevation is a sign of failed thrombolysis. Emergency catheterization should be considered to achieve reperfusion**
- **Cardiogenic shock is an additional reason for emergency catheterization. In the case of an inferior MI it is also important to consider right ventricular infarction rather than pump failure as a cause for shock. Neck vein distension with clear lungs are clinical signs of a right ventricular infarct**
- **This patient received a GP IIb/IIIa inhibitor in the catheterization laboratory prior to stent placement. This is contraindicated in the setting of full-dose thrombolytic but bleeding risk is acceptable after half-dose fibrinolytic treatment**

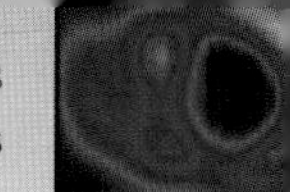

Abbreviations

Cardiovascular conditions and terminology

AAA	Abdominal aortic aneurysm
ACS	Acute coronary syndrome
AV	Atrioventricular
CAD	Coronary artery disease
CHD	Coronary heart disease
CHF	Congestive heart failure
COPD	Chronic obstructive pulmonary disease
CV	Cardiovascular
FMD	Flow-mediated endothelium-dependent dilatation
HIT	Heparin-induced thrombocytopenia
IHD	Ischaemic heart disease
LAD	Left anterior descending
LV	Left ventricular
LVF	Left ventricular failure
MI	Myocardial infarction
MR	Mitral regurgitation
NSTEMI	Non-ST segment elevation myocardial infarction
RCA	Right coronary artery
STEMI	ST-segment elevation myocardial infarction
UA	Unstable angina

Drugs and molecules

ACE	Angiotensin converting enzyme
ADP	Adenosine diphosphate
AII	Angiotensin II
Apo	Apolipoprotein
ARB	Angiotensin receptor blocker
BMIPP	^{123}I beta-methyliodophenyl pentadecanoic acid
BNP	B-type natriuretic peptide
CK	Creatinine kinase
CK-MB	Creatinine kinase myoglobin
CRP	C-reactive protein
e-NOS	Endothelial nitric oxide synthase
FDG	Fluorodeoxyglucose
GP	Glycoprotein
HDL	High-density lipoprotein
HRT	Hormone replacement therapy
ICAM	Intracellular adhesion molecule

Il-1	Interleukin-1
Il-6	Interleukin-6
LDH	Lactate dehydrogenase
LDL	Low-density lipoprotein
LMWH	Low molecular weight heparin
Lp(a)	Lipoprotein (a)
MB	Myoglobin
MMP	Matrix metalloproteinases
NO	Nitric oxide
NSAID	Nonsteroidal anti-inflammatory drug
NT-proBNP	N-Terminal pro-Brain Natriuretic Peptide
PAF	Platelet activating factor
PDGF	Platelet-derived growth factor
TNF	Tumour necrosis factor
TnI	Troponin I
TnT	Troponin T
TXA_2	Thromboxane A_2
UFH	Unfractionated heparin
VCAM	Vascular cell adhesion molecule

Examinations and procedures

aPTT	Activated partial thromboplastin time
CABG	Coronary artery bypass graft
CPR	Cardio-pulmonary resuscitation
ECG	Electrocardiogram
hsCRP	High-sensitivity C-reactive protein
IABP	Intra-aortic balloon pumping
METS	Metabolic equivalents
MPI	Myocardial perfusion imaging
PCI	Percutaneous coronary intervention

Organizations

ACC	American College of Cardiology
ACCP	American College of Chest Physicians
AHA	American Heart Association
CCS	Canadian Cardiovascular Society
ESC	European Society of Cardiology
FDA	Food and Drug Administration

Other

CI	Confidence interval
DC	Direct current
EMS	Emergency medical services

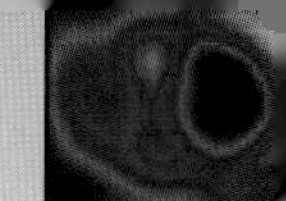

iv	Intravenous
NSF	National service framework
OR	Odds ratio
RR	Risk reduction

Trials

4S	Scandinavian Simvastatin Survival Study
A to Z	Aggrastat to Zocor
ACADEMIC	Azithromycin in Coronary Artery Disease: Elimination of Myocardial Infection with Chlamydia
ACES	Azithromycin in Coronary Events Study
ACTION	A Coronary disease Trial Investigating Outcome with Nifedipine gastrointestinal therapeutic system
AFCAPS/TexCAPS	Air Force/Texas Coronary Atherosclerosis Prevention Study
AMISTAD	Acute Myocardial Infarction Study of Adenosine
ANTIBIO	Antibiotic Therapy after Acute Myocardial Infarction
ASCOT	Anglo-Scandinavian Cardiac Outcomes Trial
ASCOT-LLA	Anglo-Scandinavian Cardiac Outcomes Trial – Lipid Lowering Arm
ASSENT	Assessment of the Safety and Efficacy of a New Thrombolytic
AZACS	Azithromycin in Acute Coronary Syndrome
CAPTIM	Comparison of Angioplasty and Prehospital Thrombolysis in Acute Myocardial Infarction
CAPTURE	Randomised Placebo-controlled Trial of Abciximab Before and During Coronary Intervention in Refractory Unstable Angina
CARE	Cholesterol and Recurrent Events Trial
CCS	Chinese Cardiac Study
CDP	Coronary Drug Project
CLARITY-TIMI	Clopidogrel as Adjunctive Reperfusion Therapy-Thrombolysis in Myocardial Infarction
COMMIT	Comprehensive Multidisciplinary Intervention Trial for Regression of Coronary Artery Disease
CONSENSUS	Cooperative North Scandinavian Enalapril Survival Study

CREDO	Clopidogrel for the Reduction of Events During Observation
CRUSADE	Can Rapid Risk Stratification of Unstable Angina Patients Suppress Adverse Outcomes With Early Implementation of the ACC/AHA Guidelines?
CURE	Clopidogrel in Unstable Angina to prevent Recurrent Events
DANAMI-2	Danish Multi-centre Trial in Acute Myocardial Infarction-2
ER-TIMI	Early Retavase-Thrombolysis in Myocardial Infarction
ESSENCE	Efficacy and Safety of Subcutaneous Enoxaparin in Non-Q-wave Coronary Events
EUROPA	European Trial on Reduction of Cardiac Events with Perindopril in Stable Coronary Artery Disease
FRAXIS	Fraxiparine in Ischemic Syndromes
FRIC	Fragmin In Unstable Coronary Artery Disease
FRISC	Fragmin During Instability in Coronary Artery Disease
GISSI-3	Gruppo Italiano per lo Studio della Sopravvivenza nell'Infarto Miocardico III (lisinopril and transdermal glyceryl trinitrate)
GRACE	Global Registry of Acute Coronary Events
GUSTO	Global Utilization of Strategies to Open Occluded Coronary Arteries
HINT	Holland Interuniversity Nifedipine/metoprolol Trial
HOPE	Heart Outcomes Prevention Evaluation Study
HPS	Heart Protection Study
ICTUS	Invasive versus Conservative Treatment in Unstable Coronary Syndromes
INTERACT	Integrilin and Enoxaparin Randomized Assessment of Acute Coronary Syndrome Treatment
INTERCEPT	Incomplete Infarction Trial of European Research Collaborators Evaluating Prognosis Post-Thrombolysis
INTERHEART	Global Study of Risk Factors in Acute Myocardial Infarction
IONA	Impact of Nicorandil in Angina

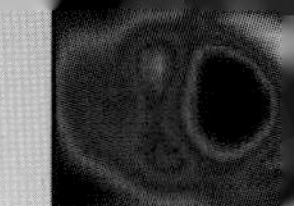

ISAR-3	Intracoronary Stenting and Antibiotic Regimen 3
ISAR-COOL	Intracoronary Stenting with Antithrombotic Regiment Cooling-Off
ISIS-4	Fourth International Study of Infarct Survival
LIPID	Long-term Intervention with Pravastatin in Ischaemic heart Disease
MINAP	Myocardial Infarction National Audit Project
MIRACL	Myocardial Ischemia Reduction with Aggressive Cholesterol Lowering
OASIS	Organization to Assess Strategies for Ischemic Syndromes
PEACE	Prevention of Events with Angiotensin Converting Enzyme Inhibition
PRISM	Platelet Receptor Inhibition in Ischemic Syndrome Management
PRISM-PLUS	Platelet Receptor Inhibition in Ischemic Syndrome Management in Patients Limited by Unstable Signs and Symptoms
PROACTIVE	Prospective Pioglitazone Clinical Trial in Macrovascular Events Study
PROVE IT	Pravastatin or Atorvastatin Evaluation and Infection Therapy Trial
PURSUIT	Platelet Glycoprotein IIb/IIIa in Unstable Angina: Receptor Suppression Using Integrilin Therapy
RAPID	Reteplase vs Alteplase Infusion in Acute Myocardial Infarction (or Reteplase vs Alteplase Patency Investigation During Myocardial Infarction)
REACT	Rescue Angioplasty versus Conservative Therapy or Repeat Thrombolysis Trial
REPLACE	Randomized Evaluation in PCI Linking Angiomax to Reduced Clinical Events
RESTORE	Randomized Efficacy Study of Tirofiban for Outcomes and Restenosis
REVERSAL	Reversal of Atherosclerosis with Aggressive Lipid Lowering
RISC	Research on Instability in Coronary Artery Disease
RITA	Randomized Intervention Trial of Unstable Angina

SHOCK	Should we emergently revascularize occluded coronaries for cardiogenic shock?
SMIR	Singapore Myocardial Infarction Register
SPEED	Strategies for Patency Enhancement in the Emergency Department
STAMINA	South Thames Trial of Antibiotics in Myocardial Infarction and Unstable Angina
STRATEGY	Tirofiban and Sirolimus-eluting Stent vs Abciximab and Bare-metal Stent for Acute Myocardial Infarction
SYNERGY	Superior Yield of the New Strategy of Enoxaparin, Revascularization and Glycoprotein IIb/IIIa Inhibitors
TACTICS-TIMI-18	Treat Angina With Aggrastat and Determine Cost of Therapy With Invasive or Conservative Strategy – Thrombolysis In Myocardial Infarction
TARGET	Do Tirofiban and ReoPro Give Similar Efficacy Outcomes Trial
TIMI	Thrombolysis in Myocardial Infarction
TNT	Treating to New Targets
VA-HIT	Veterans Affairs High-Density Lipoprotein Cholesterol Intervention Trial
VALIANT	Valsartan in Acute Myocardial Infarction
VANQWISH	Veterans Affairs Non-Q-Wave Infarction Strategies in Hospital
WIZARD	Weekly Intervention with Zithromax for Atherosclerosis and its Related Disorders
WOSCOPS	West of Scotland Coronary Prevention Study

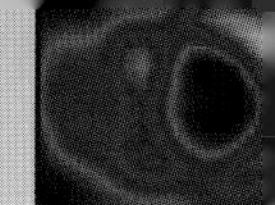

Contact information for useful organizations

American College of Cardiology
Heart House, 9111 Old Georgetown Road, Bethesda,
MD 20814-1699, USA
Tel: +1 800 253 4636, ext. 694
Fax: +1 301 897 9745
Website: http://www.acc.org

American College of Chest Physicians
3300 Dundee Road, Northbrook, Illinois 60062-2348, USA
Tel: +1 847 498 1400
Website: http://www.chestnet.org

American Heart Association
One North Franklin, Chicago, IL 60606-3412, USA
Tel: +1 312 422 3000
Website: http://www.aha.org

American Society of Echocardiography
1500 Sunday Drive, Suite 102, Raleigh, NC 27607, USA
Tel: +1 919 861 5574
Fax: +1 919 787 4916
Website: http://www.asecho.org

American Society of Hypertension
148 Madison Avenue, New York, NY 10016, USA
Tel: +1 212 696 9099
Fax: +1 212 696 0711
E-mail: ash@ash-us.org

American Society of Nuclear Cardiology
9111 Old Georgetown Road, Bethesda, MD 20814-1699, USA
Tel: +1 301 493 2360
Fax: +1 301 493 2376
E-mail: admin@asnc.org
Website: http://www.asnc.org

British Cardiac Society
9 Fitzroy Square, London W1T 5HW, UK
Tel: +44 (0)20 7383 3887
Fax: +44 (0)20 7388 0903
Website: http://www.bcs.com

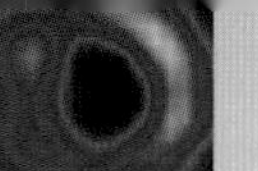

British Heart Foundation
14 Fitzhardinge Street, London W1H 6DH, UK
Tel: +44 (0)20 7935 0185
Fax: +44 (0)20 7486 5820
E-mail: internet@bhf.org.uk
Website: http://www.bhf.org.uk

British Nuclear Cardiology Society
c/o Department of Nuclear Medicine, Royal Brompton Hospital, Sydney Street, London SW3 6NP, UK
Tel: +44 (0)20 7351 8884
Fax: +44 (0)20 7351 8885
Website: http://www.bncs.org.uk

Canadian Cardiovascular Society
222 Queen Street, Suite 1403, Orrawa, Ontario, K1P 5V9, Canada
Tel: +1 613 569 3407
Fax: +1 613 569 6574
E-mail: ccsinfo@ccs.ca
Website: http://www.ccs.ca

European Atherosclerosis Society
Secretary, Dr Sebastiano Calandra, Sezione di Patologia Generale, Dipartimento di Scienze Biomediche, Universita di Modena e Reggio Emilia, Via Campi 287, I-41100 Modena, Italy
Tel: +39 059 2055 423
Fax: +39 059 2055 426
Website: http://www.elsevier.com/inca

European Society of Cardiology
The European Heart House, 2035 Route des Colles B.P. 179 – Les Templiers, FR-06903 Sophia Antipolis, France
Tel: +33 4 92 94 76 00
Fax: +33 4 92 94 76 01
E-mail: webmaster@escardio.org
Website: http://www.escardio.org

European Society of Hypertension
Institute of Clinical Experimental Medicine, Dept of Preventive Cardiology, Videnska 1958/9. 140 21 Prague 4. Czech Republic
Tel: +420 2 617 11 399
Fax: +420 2 617 10 666
E-mail: info@eshonline.org
Website: http://www.eshonline.org

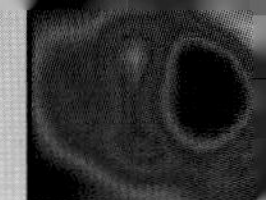

Heart UK
7 North Road, Maidenhead, Berkshire SL6 1PE, UK
Tel: +44 (0)1628 628 638
Fax: +44 (0)1628 628 698
E-mail: ask@heartuk.org.uk
Website: http://www.heartuk.org.uk

National Heart Lung and Blood Institute
NHLBI Health Information Center, PO Box 30105, Bethesda, MD 20824-0105, USA
Tel: +1 301 592 8573
Fax: +1 301 592 8563
Website: http://www.nhi.org

Primary Care Cardiovascular Society
36 Berrymede Road, London W4 5JD, UK
Tel: +44 (0)20 8994 8775
Fax: +44 (0)20 8742 2130
E-mail: office@pccs.org.uk
Website: http://www.pccs.org.uk

Society for Cardiovascular Angiography and Interventions
9111 Old Georgetown Road, Bethesda, MD 20814, USA
Tel: +1 301 581 3450
Fax: +1 301 581 3408
E-mail: info@scai.org
Website: http://www.scai.org

Society of Geriatric Cardiology
Heart House, 9111 Old Georgetown Road, Bethesda, MD 20814-1699, USA
Tel: +1 301 581 3449
Fax: +1 301 581 3456
Website: http://www.sgcard.org

World Heart Federation
5, avenue du Mail, 1205 Geneva, Switzerland
Tel: +41 22 807 03 20
Fax: +41 22 807 03 39
E-mail: admin@worldheart.org
Website: http://www.worldheart.org

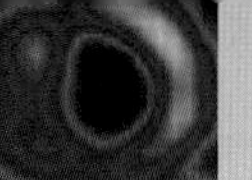

References

1. Committee on the Management of Patients with Unstable Angina. ACC/AHA guidelines for the management of patients with unstable angina and non-ST-segment elevation myocardial infarction. J Am Coll Cardiol 2000;36:970–1062.
2. Fox KAA, Goodman SG, Klein W, et al. Management of acute coronary syndromes. Variations in practice and outcome. Findings from the Global Registry of Acute Coronary Events (GRACE). Eur Heart J 2002;23:1177–1189.
3. The Joint European Society of Cardiology/American College of Cardiology Committee. Myocardial infarction redefined – A consensus document of the Joint European Society of Cardiology/American College of Cardiology Committee for the redefinition of myocardial infarction. Eur Heart J 2000;21:1502–1513.
4. French JK, White HD. Clinical implications of the new definition of myocardial infarction. Heart 2004;90:99–106.
5. American Heart Association. Heart Disease and Stroke Statistics – 2005 Update. Dallas, Texas: American Heart Association, 2005.
6. Murphy NF, MacIntyre K, Capewell S, et al. Hospital discharge rates for suspected acute coronary syndromes between 1990 and 2000: population based analysis. BMJ 2004;328:1413–1414.
7. Agency for Health Care Policy and Research, National Heart, Lung and Blood Institute. Unstable angina: diagnosis and management, clinical practice guideline no. 10. Rockville, MD: US Department of Health and Human Services, Public Health Service, AHCPR Publication no. 94-0602, March 1994.
8. Hasdai D, Behar S, Wallentin L, et al. The Euro heart survey of acute coronary syndromes. Eur Heart J 2002;23:1190–1201.
9. Timmis A. Acute coronary syndromes: risk stratification. Heart 2000;83:241–246.
10. Barakat K, Wilkinson P, Deaner A, et al. How should age affect management of acute myocardial infarction? A prospective cohort study. Lancet 1999;353:955–959.
11. Goldberg RJ, Currie K, White K, et al. The Global Registry of Acute Coronary Events GRACE. Am J Cardiol 2004;93:288–293.
12. Bonetti PO, Lerman LO, Lerman A. Endothelial dysfunction. A marker of atherosclerotic risk. Arterioscler Thromb Vasc Biol 2003;23:168–175.
13. MacIsaac AI, Thomas JD, Topol EJ. Toward the quiescent coronary plaque. JACC 1993;22:1228–1241.
14. Davies MJ. The role of plaque pathology in coronary thrombosis. Clin Cardiol 1997;20(Suppl 1):1-2-1-7.
15. Theroux P, Fuster V. Acute coronary syndromes. Unstable angina and non-Q-wave myocardial infarction. Circulation 1998;97:1195–1206.
16. Libby P. Molecular basis of the acute coronary syndromes. Circulation 1995;91:2844–2850.
17. Pignalberi C, Patti G, Chimenti C, et al. Role of different determinants of psychological distress in acute coronary syndromes. J Am Coll Cardiol 1998;32:613–619.
18. Jones CB, Sane DC, Herrington DM. Matrix metalloproteinases: a review of their structure and role in acute coronary syndrome. Cardiovasc Res 2003;59:812–823.
19. Schachter M. Lipid lowering drugs, inflammation and cardiovascular disease. Br J Diabetes Vasc Dis 2003;3:178–182.
20. Ross R. Atherosclerosis – an inflammatory disease. N Engl J Med 1999;340:115–126.
21. Hansson GK. Inflammation, atherosclerosis, and coronary artery disease. N Engl J Med 2005;352:1685–1695.
22. Buffon A, Biasucci LM, Liuzzo G, et al. Widespread inflammation in unstable angina. N Engl J Med 2002;347:5–12.
23. Ridker PM, Rifai N, Rose L, et al. Comparison of C-reactive protein and low-density lipoprotein cholesterol levels in the predicition of first cardiovascular events. N Engl J Med 2002;347:1557–1565.
24. Ridker PM. Clinical application of C-reactive protein for cardiovascular disease detection and prevention. Circulation 2003;107:363–369.
25. Galvani M, Ottani F, Oltrona, et al. N-terminal pro-brain natriuretic peptide on admission has prognostic value across the whole spectrum of acute coronary syndromes. Circulation 2004;110:128–134.
26. Rupprecht HJ. Adenosine diphosphate receptor antagonists: from pharmacology to clinical practice. Eur Heart J 2000;2(Suppl E):E1–E5.
27. Udelson JE, Beshansky JR, Ballin DS, et al. Myocardial perfusion imaging for evaluation and triage of patients with suspected acute cardiac ischemia: a randomized controlled trial. JAMA 2002;288:2693–2700.
28. Braunwald E, Antman EM, Beasley JW, et al. ACC/AHA 2002 guideline update for the management of patients with unstable angina and non-ST-segment elevation myocardial infarction–summary article: a report of the American College of Cardiology/American Heart Association task force on practice guidelines (Committee on the Management of Patients With Unstable Angina). J Am Coll Cardiol 2002;40:1366–1374.
29. Erhardt L, Herlitz J, Bossaert L, et al. Task force on the management of chest pain. Eur Heart J 2002;23:1153–1176.
30. Welch RD, Zalenski RJ, Frederick PD, et al. Prognostic value of a normal or non-specific initial electrocardiogram in acute myocardial infarction. JAMA 2001;286:1977–1984.
31. Yeghiazarians Y, Braunstein JB, Askari A, Stone PH. Unstable angina pectoris. N Engl J Med 2000;342:101–112.
32. Stone PH, Thompson B, Zaret BI, et al. Factors associated with failure of medical therapy in patients with unstable angina and non-Q-wave myocardial infarction: a TIMI IIIB database study. Eur Heart J 1999;20:1084–1093.
33. Savonitto S, Ardissino D, Granger CB, et al. Prognostic value of the admission electrocardiogram in acute coronary syndromes. JAMA 1999;281:707–713.
34. von Arnim T, Gerbig HW, Krawietz W, et al. Prognostic implications of transient–predominantly silent–ischaemia in patients with unstable angina pectoris. Eur Heart J 1988;9:435–440.
35. Bertrand ME, Simoons ML, Fox KAA, et al. Management of acute coronary syndromes in patients presenting without persistent ST-segment elevation. The Task Force on the Management of Acute Coronary Syndromes of the European Society of Cardiology. Eur Heart J 2002;23:1809–1840.
36. Antman EM, Cohen M, Bernink PJLM, et al. The TIMI risk score for unstable angina/non-ST elevation MI. JAMA 2000;284:835–842.
37. De Araujo Goncalves P, Ferreira J, Aguiar C, Seabra-Gomes R. TIMI, PURSUIT, and GRACE: sustained prognostic value and interaction with revascularization in NSTE-ACS. Eur Heart J 2005:26:805–872.
38. Reader GS. Management of acute myocardial infarction: risk stratification after thrombolytic therapy. In: Murphy JG, editor. Mayo Clinic Cardiology Review. Armonk, NY: Futura Publishing, 1997; Chapter 14, pp. 139–146.
39. Ferreiros ER, Boissonnet CP, Pizarro R, et al. Independent prognostic value of elevated C-reactive protein in unstable angina. Circulation 1999;100:1958–1963.
40. Ridker PM, Brown NJ, Vaughan DE, et al. Established and emerging plasma biomarkers in the prediction of first atherothrombotic events. Circulation 2004;109(Suppl IV):IV-6–IV-19.

41. Sadanandan S, Cannon CP, Chekuri K, et al. Association of elevated B-Type natriuretic peptide levels with angiographic findings among patients with unstable angina and non-ST segment elevation myocardial infarction. J Am Coll Cardiol 2004;44:564–568.
42. Gibbons RJ, Balady GJ, Bricker JT, et al. ACC/AHA guideline update for exercise testing: summary article. Circulation 2002;106:1883–1892.
43. Valeur N, Clemmensen P, Saunamaki K, Grande P, for the DANAMI-2 investigators. The prognostic value of pre-discharge exercise testing after myocardial infarction with either primary PCI or fibrinolysis: a DANAMI-2 sub-study. Eur Heart J 2005:26:119–127.
44. Loong CY, Anagnostopoulos C. Diagnosis of coronary artery disease by radionuclide myocardial perfusion imaging. Heart 2004;90 Suppl 5:v2–v9.
45. Wackers FJ, Lie KI, Liem KL, et al. Potential value of thallium-201 scintigraphy as a means of selecting patients for the coronary care unit. Br Heart J 1979;41:111–117.
46. Varetto T, Cantalupi D, Altieri A, Orlandi C. Emergency room technetium-99m sestamibi imaging to rule out acute myocardial ischemic events in patients with nondiagnostic electrocardiograms. J Am Coll Cardiol 1993;22:1804–1808.
47. Wackers FJ, Brown KA, Heller GV, et al. American Society of Nuclear Cardiology position statement on radionuclide imaging in patients with suspected acute ischemic syndromes in the emergency department or chest pain center. J Nucl Cardiol 2002;9:246–250.
48. Bilodeau L, Theroux P, Gregoire J, et al. Technetium-99m sestamibi tomography in patients with spontaneous chest pain: correlations with clinical, electrocardiographic and angiographic findings. J Am Coll Cardiol 1991;18:1684–1691.
49. Hilton TC, Thompson RC, Williams HJ, et al. Technetium-99m sestamibi myocardial perfusion imaging in the emergency room evaluation of chest pain. J Am Coll Cardiol 1994;23:1016–1022.
50. Kontos MC, Jesse RL, Schmidt KL, et al. Value of acute rest sestamibi perfusion imaging for evaluation of patients admitted to the emergency department with chest pain. J Am Coll Cardiol 1997;30:976–982.
51. Kontos MC, Jesse RL, Anderson FP, et al. Comparison of myocardial perfusion imaging and cardiac troponin I in patients admitted to the emergency department with chest pain. Circulation 1999;99:2073–2078.
52. Heller GV, Stowers SA, Hendel RC, et al. Clinical value of acute rest technetium-99m tetrofosmin tomographic myocardial perfusion imaging in patients with acute chest pain and nondiagnostic electrocardiograms. J Am Coll Cardiol 1998;31:1011–1017.
53. Radensky PW, Hilton TC, Fulmer H, et al. Potential cost effectiveness of initial myocardial perfusion imaging for assessment of emergency department patients with chest pain. Am J Cardiol 1997;9:595–599.
54. Duca MD, Giri S, Wu AH, et al. Comparison of acute rest myocardial perfusion imaging and serum markers of myocardial injury in patients with chest pain syndromes. J Nucl Cardiol 1999;6:570–576.
55. Stratmann HG, Tamesis BR, Younis LT, et al. Prognostic value of predischarge dipyridamole technetium 99m sestamibi myocardial tomography in medically treated patients with unstable angina. Am Heart J 1995;130:734–740.
56. Klocke FJ, Baird MG, Lorell BH, et al. ACC/AHA/ASNC guidelines for the clinical use of cardiac radionuclide imaging–executive summary: a report of the American College of Cardiology/American Heart Association Task Force on Practice Guidelines (ACC/AHA/ASNC Committee to Revise the 1995 Guidelines for the Clinical Use of Cardiac Radionuclide Imaging). J Am Coll Cardiol 2003;42:1318–1333.
57. Van de Werf F, Ardissino D, Betriu A, et al. Management of acute myocardial infarction in patients presenting with ST-segment elevation. The Task Force on the Management of Acute Myocardial Infarction of the European Society of Cardiology. Eur Heart J 2003;24:28–66.
58. Antman EM, Anbe DT, Armstrong PW, et al. ACC/AHA guidelines for the management of patients with ST-elevation myocardial infarction: A report of the American College of Cardiology/American Heart Association Task Force on Practice Guidelines (Committee to Revise the 1999 Guidelines for the Management of patients with acute myocardial infarction). J Am Coll Cardiol 2004;44:E1–E211.
59. Madsen JK, Grande P, Saunamaki K, et al. Danish multicenter randomized study of invasive versus conservative treatment in patients with inducible ischemia after thrombolysis in acute myocardial infarction (DANAMI). DANish trial in Acute Myocardial Infarction. Circulation 1997;96:748–755.
60. Anagnostopoulos C, Harbinson M, Kelion A, et al. Procedure guidelines for radionuclide myocardial perfusion imaging. Heart 2004;90 Suppl 1:i1–10.
61. Heller GV, Brown KA, Landin RJ, Haber SB. Safety of early intravenous dipyridamole technetium 99m sestamibi SPECT myocardial perfusion imaging after uncomplicated first myocardial infarction. Early Post MI IV Dipyridamole Study (EPIDS). Am Heart J 1997;134:105–111.
62. Brown KA, Heller GV, Landin RS, et al. Early dipyridamole (99m)Tc-sestamibi single photon emission computed tomographic imaging 2 to 4 days after acute myocardial infarction predicts in-hospital and postdischarge cardiac events: comparison with submaximal exercise imaging. Circulation 1999;100:2060–2066.
63. Kroll D, Farah W, McKendall GR, et al. Prognostic value of stress-gated Tc-99m sestamibi SPECT after acute myocardial infarction. Am J Cardiol 2001;87:381–386.
64. DePuey EG, Rozanski A. Using gated technetium-99m-sestamibi SPECT to characterize fixed myocardial defects as infarct or artifact. J Nucl Med 1995;36:952–955.
65. Loh IK, Charuzi Y, Beeder C, et al. Early diagnosis of nontransmural myocardial infarction by two-dimensional echocardiography. Am Heart J 1982;104(5 Pt 1):963–968.
66. Sabia P, Afrookteh A, Touchstone DA, et al. Value of regional wall motion abnormality in the emergency room diagnosis of acute myocardial infarction. A prospective study using two-dimensional echocardiography. Circulation 1991;84(3 Suppl):I85–I92.
67. Mahmarian JJ, Shaw LJ, Olszewski GH, et al. Adenosine sestamibi SPECT post-infarction evaluation (INSPIRE) trial: A randomized, prospective multicenter trial evaluating the role of adenosine Tc-99m sestamibi SPECT for assessing risk and therapeutic outcomes in survivors of acute myocardial infarction. J Nucl Cardiol 2004;11:458–469.
68. Kawai Y, Tsukamoto E, Nozaki Y, et al. Significance of reduced uptake of iodinated fatty acid analogue for the evaluation of patients with acute chest pain. J Am Coll Cardiol 2001;38:1888–1894.
69. Kaddoura S. Echo Made Easy. Edinburgh: Churchill Livingstone, 2002.
70. Fox KF. Investigation and management of chest pain. Heart 2005:91:105–110.
71. Patel DJ, Gomma AH, Knight CJ, et al. Why is recurrent myocardial ischaemia a predictor of adverse outcome in unstable angina? Eur Heart J 2001;22:1991–1996.
72. Chen L, Chester MR, Redwood S, et al. Angiographic stenosis progression and coronary events in patients with 'stabilized' unstable angina. Circulation 1995;91:2319–2324.

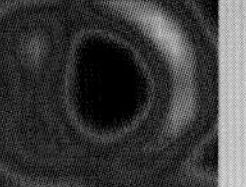

73. Silva JA, Escobar A, Collins TJ, et al. Unstable angina. A comparison of angioscopic findings between diabetic and nondiabetic patients. Circulation 1995:92:1731–1736.
74. Mukherjee D, Fang J, Chetcuti S, et al. Impact of combination evidence-based medical therapy on mortality in patients with acute coronary syndromes. Circulation 2004;109:745–749.
75. Mukherjee D, Fang J, Kline-Rogers E, et al. Impact of combination evidence based medical treatment in patients with acute coronary syndromes in various TIMI risk groups. Heart 2005;91:381–382.
76. Gluckman TJ, Sachdev M, Schulman SP, Blumenthal RS. A simplified approach to the management of non-ST-segment elevation acute coronary syndromes. JAMA 2005;293:349–357.
77. Purcell H, Patel DJ, Mulcahy D, Fox K. Nicorandil. In: Messerli FH, editor. Cardiovascular drug therapy, 2nd edition. Philadelphia: WB Saunders Co, 1996; Chapter 178, pp 1638–1645.
78. Patel DJ, Purcell HJ, Fox KM on behalf of the CESAR 2 investigation. Cardioprotection by opening of the K_{ATP} channel in unstable angina. Is this a clinical manifestation of myocardial preconditioning? Results of a randomized study with nicorandil. Eur Heart J 1999;20:51–57.
79. The IONA Study Group. Effect of nicorandil on coronary events in patients with stable angina: the Impact Of Nicorandil in Angina (IONA) randomised trial. Lancet 2002;359:1269–1275.
80. Lopez Sendon J, Swedberg K, McMurray J, et al. Expert consensus document on B-adrenergic receptor blockers. Eur Heart J 2004;25:1341–1362.
81. Freemantle N, Cleland J, Young P, et al. ß blockade after myocardial infarction: systematic review of meta regression analysis. BMJ 1999;318:1730–1737.
82. Gottlieb SS, McCarter RJ. Comparative effects of three beta blockers (atenolol, metoprolol, and propranolol) on survival after acute myocardial infarction. Am J Cardiol 2001;87:823–826.
83. Goldstein S. Beta-blocking drugs and coronary heart disease. Cardiovasc Drugs Ther 1997;11:219–225.
84. Thadani U. Medical therapy of stable angina pectoris. Cardiol Clin 1991;9:73–87.
85. Purcell H, Waller DG, Fox K. Calcium antagonists in cardiovascular disease. Br J Clin Pract 1989;43:369–379.
86. Pitt B, Byington RP, Furberg CD, et al. Effect of amlodipine on the progression of atherosclerosis and the occurrence of clinical events. PREVENT investigators. Circulation 2000;102:1503–1510.
87. Held PH, Yusuf S, Furberg CD. Calcium channel blockers in acute myocardial infarction and unstable angina: an overview. BMJ 1989;299:1187–1192.
88. Lubsen J, Tijssen JG. Efficacy of nifedipine and metoprolol in the early treatment of unstable angina in the coronary care unit: findings from the Holland Interuniversity Nifedipine/metoprolol Trial (HINT). Am J Cardiol 1987;60:18A–25A.
89. Antman EM, Beasley JW, Califf RM, et al. ACC/AHA Guidelines for the management of patients with unstable angina and non-ST-segment elevation myocardial infarction. J Am Coll Cardiol 2000;36:970–1062.
90. Blood Pressure Lowering Treatment Trialists' Collaboration. Effects of different blood-pressure-lowering regimens on major cardiovascular events: results of prospectively-designed overviews of randomised trials. Lancet 2003;362:1527–1535.
91. Poole-Wilson PA, Lubsen J, Kirwan BA, et al. Effect of long-acting nifedipine on mortality and cardiovascular morbidity in patients with stable angina requiring treatment (ACTION trial): randomised controlled trial. Lancet 2004;364:849–857.
92. Boden WE, van Gilst WH, Scheldewaert RG, et al. Diltiazem in acute myocardial infarction treated with thrombolytic agents: a randomised placebo-controlled trial. Lancet 2000;335:1751–1756.
93. Antithrombotic Trialists' Collaboration. Collaborative meta-analysis of randomised trials of antiplatelet therapy for prevention of death, myocardial infarction, and stroke in high risk patients. BMJ 2002;324:71–86.
94. Patrono C, Coller B, Dalen JE, et al. Platelet-active drugs: The relationships among dose, effectiveness, and side-effects. Chest 2001;119:39S–63S.
95. Patrono C, Bachmann F, Baigent C, et al. Expert consensus document on the use of antiplatelet agents. Eur Heart J 2004;25:166–181.
96. Guyatt G, Albers G, Schunemann H (eds). The Seventh ACCP Conference in Antithrombotic and Thrombolytic Therapy: evidence-based guidelines. Chest 2004;126(3 Suppl):228S–252S.
97. Peters RJG, Mehta SR, Fox KAA, et al. Effects of aspirin dose when used alone or in combination with clopidogrel in patients with acute coronary syndromes. Circulation 2003;108:1682–1687.
98. Cannon CP. Oval platelet glycoprotein IIb/IIIa blockers. In: Ferguson JJ, Chronos NAF, Harrington RA, editors. Antiplatelet Therapy in Clinical Practice. London: Martin Dunitz, 2000; Chapter 10, pp. 163–177.
99. Folts JD, Schafer AI, Loscalzo J, et al. A perspective on the potential problems with aspirin as an antithrombotic agent: a comparison of studies in an animal model with clinical trials. J Am Coll Cardiol 1999;33:296–303.
100. Yusuf S, Zhao F, Mehta SR, et al. Effects of clopidogrel in addition to aspirin in patients with acute coronary syndromes without ST-segment elevation. N Engl J Med 2001;345(7):494–502.
101. Mehta SR, Yusuf S, Peters RJ, et al. Effects of pretreatment with clopidogrel and aspirin followed by long-term therapy in patients undergoing percutaneous coronary intervention: the PCI-CURE study. Lancet 2001;358:527–533.
102. Steinhubl SR, Berger PB, Mann JT 3rd, et al; CREDO Investigators. Early and sustained dual oral antiplatelet therapy following percutaneous intervention: a randomized controlled trial. JAMA 2002;288:2411–20.
103. Braunwald E, Antman EM, Beasley JW, et al. ACC/AHA guideline update for the management of patients with unstable angina and non-ST-segment elevation myocardial infarction–2002: summary article: a report of the American College of Cardiology/American Heart Association Task Force on Practice Guidelines (Committee on the Management of Patients With Unstable Angina). Circulation 2002;106:1893–1900.
104. Harrington RA, Becker RC, Ezekowitz M, et al. Antithrombotic therapy for coronary artery disease: the Seventh ACCP Conference on Antithrombotic and Thrombolytic Therapy. Chest 2004;126(3 Suppl):513S–548S.
105. Silber S, Albertsson P, Aviles FF, et al. Guidelines for percutaneous coronary interventions: the task force for percutaneous coronary interventions of the European Society of Cardiology. Eur Heart J 2005;26:804–847.
106. Popma JJ, Berger P, Ohman EM, et al. Antithrombotic therapy during percutaneous coronary intervention: the Seventh ACCP Conference on Antithrombotic and Thrombolytic Therapy. Chest 2004;126(3 Suppl):576S–599S.
107. Wiviott SD, Antman EM. Clopidogrel resistance: a new chapter in a fast-moving story. Circulation 2004;109:3064–3067.
108. Boeynaems JM, van Giezen H, Savi P, et al. P2Y receptor antagonists in thrombosis. Curr Opin Invest Drugs 2005;6:275–282.
109. Falk E, Shah PK, Fuster V. Coronary plaque disruption. Circulation 1995;92:657–671.
110. Gibson CM, Cannon CP, Murphy SA, et al. Relationship of TIMI myocardial perfusion grade to mortality after administration of thrombolytic drugs. Circulation 2000;101:125–130.
111. Gibson CM, Cohen DJ, Cohen EA, et al. Effect of eptifibatide on coronary flow reserve following coronary stent implantation (an ESPRIT substudy). Enhanced suppression of the platelet IIb/IIIa receptor with integrilin therapy. Am J Cardiol 2001;87:1293–1295.

112. Kong DF, Califf RM, Miller DP, et al. Clinical outcomes of therapeutic agents that block the platelet glycoprotein IIb/IIIa integrin in ischemic heart disease. Circulation 1998;98:2829–2835.
113. Phillips DR, Scarborough RM. Clinical pharmacology of eptifibatide. Am J Cardiol 1997;80:11B–20B.
114. The PURSUIT Trial Investigators. Inhibition of platelet glycoprotein IIb/IIIa with eptifibatide in patients with acute coronary syndromes. N Engl J Med 1998;339:436–443.
115. The RESTORE Investigators. Effects of platelet glycoprotein IIb/IIIa blockade with tirofiban on adverse cardiac events in patients with unstable angina or acute myocardial infarction undergoing coronary angioplasty. Circulation 1997;96:1445–1453.
116. The Platelet Receptor Inhibition in Ischemic Syndrome Management (PRISM) Study Investigators. A comparison of aspirin plus tirofiban with aspirin plus heparin for unstable angina. N Engl J Med 1998;338:1498–1505.
117. The Platelet Receptor Inhibition in Ischemic Syndrome Management in Patients Limited by Unstable Signs and Symptoms (PRISM-PLUS) Study Investigators. Inhibition of the platelet glycoprotein IIb/IIIa receptor with tirofiban in unstable angina and non-Q-wave myocardial infarction. N Engl J Med 1998;338:1488–1497.
118. Simoons ML. Effect of glycoprotein IIb/IIIa receptor blocker abciximab on outcome in patients with acute coronary syndromes without early coronary revascularisation: the GUSTO IV-ACS randomised trial. Lancet 2001;357:1915–1924.
119. Boersma E, Harrington RA, Moliterno DJ, et al. Platelet glycoprotein IIb/IIIa inhibitors in acute coronary syndromes: a meta-analysis of all major randomised clinical trials. Lancet 2002;359:189–198.
120. Karvouni E, Katritsis DG, Ioannidis JPA. Intravenous glycoprotein IIb/IIIa receptor antagonists reduce mortality after percutaneous coronary interventions. J Am Coll Cardiol 2003;41:26–32.
121. The EPISTENT Investigators. Randomised placebo-controlled and balloon-angioplasty-controlled trial to assess safety of coronary stenting with use of platelet glycoprotein-IIb/IIIa blockade. Evaluation of Platelet IIb/IIIa Inhibitor for Stenting. Lancet 1998;352:87–92.
122. ESPRIT Investigators, Enhanced Suppression on the Platelet IIb/IIIa Receptor with Integrilin Therapy. Novel dosing regimen of eptifibatide in planned coronary stent implantation (ESPRIT): a randomised, placebo-controlled trial. Lancet 2000;356:2037–2044.
123. Topol EJ, Moliterno DJ, Herrmann HC, et al. Comparison of two platelet glycoprotein IIb/IIIa inhibitors, tirofiban and abciximab, for the prevention of ischemic events with percutaneous coronary revascularization. N Engl J Med 2001;344:1888–1894.
124. Brown DL, Fann CS, Chang CJ. Meta-analysis of effectiveness and safety of abciximab versus eptifibatide or tirofiban in percutaneous coronary intervention. Am J Cardiol 2001;87:537–541.
125. Moliterno DJ, Yakubov SJ, DiBattiste PM, et al. Outcomes at 6 months for the direct comparison of tirofiban and abciximab during percutaneous coronary revascularisation with stent placement: the TARGET follow-up study. Lancet 2002;360:355–360.
126. Valgimigli M, Percoco G, Malagutti P, et al. Tirofiban and sirolimus-eluting stent vs abciximab and bare-metal stent for acute myocardial infarction: a randomized trial. JAMA 2005;293:2109–2117.
127. Lincoff AM, Califf RM, Anderson KM, et al. Evidence for prevention of death and myocardial infarction with platelet membrane glycoprotein IIb/IIIa receptor blockade by abciximab (c7E3 Fab) among patients with unstable angina undergoing percutaneous coronary revascularization. EPIC Investigators. Evaluation of 7E3 in Preventing Ischemic Complications. J Am Coll Cardiol 1997;30:149–156.
128. The CAPTURE Investigators. Randomised placebo-controlled trial of abciximab before and during coronary intervention in refractory unstable angina: the CAPTURE study. Lancet 1997;349:1429–1435.
129. Boersma E, Akkerhuis KM, Theroux P, et al. Platelet glycoprotein IIb/IIIa receptor inhibition in non-ST-elevation acute coronary syndromes: early benefit during medical treatment only, with additional protection during percutaneous coronary intervention. Circulation 1999;100:2045–2048.
130. Hamm CW, Heeschen C, Goldmann B, et al; The c7E3 Fab Antiplatelet Therapy in Unstable Refractory Angina (CAPTURE) Study Investigators. Benefit of abciximab in patients with refractory unstable angina in relation to serum troponin T levels. N Engl J Med 1999;340:1623–1629.
131. Heeschen C, Hamm CW, Goldmann B, et al. Troponin concentrations for stratification of patients with acute coronary syndromes in relation to therapeutic efficacy of tirofiban. PRISM Study Investigators. Platelet Receptor Inhibition in Ischemic Syndrome Management. Lancet 1999;354:1757–1762.
132. Peterson ED, Pollack J, Charles V, et al. Early use of glycoprotein IIb/IIIa inhibitors in non-ST-elevation acute myocardial infarction: observations from the National Registry of Myocardial Infarction 4. J Am Coll Cardiol 2003;42:45–53.
133. Braunwald E, Antman EM, Beasley JW, et al. ACC/AHA guideline update for the management of patients with unstable angina and non-ST-segment elevation myocardial infarction: a report of the American College of Cardiology/American Heart Association task force on practice guidelines (Committee on the Management of Patients With Unstable Angina). Bethesda, MD: American College of Cardiology and American Heart Association, Inc, 2002. Available at: http://www.acc.org/clinical/guidelines/unstable/unstable.pdf.
134. Theroux P, Ouimet H, McCans J, et al. Aspirin, heparin, or both to treat acute unstable angina. N Engl J Med 1988;319:1105–1111.
135. Theroux P, Waters D, Qiu S, et al. Aspirin versus heparin to prevent myocardial infarction during the acute phase of unstable angina. Circulation 1993;88(5 Pt 1):2045–2048.
136. Theroux P, Waters D, Lam J, et al. Reactivation of unstable angina after the discontinuation of heparin. N Engl J Med 1992;327:141–145.
137. Oler A, Whooley MA, Oler J, Grady D. Adding heparin to aspirin reduces the incidence of myocardial infarction and death in patients with unstable angina. A meta-analysis. JAMA 1996;276:811–815.
138. The RISC Group. Risk of myocardial infarction and death during treatment with low dose aspirin and intravenous heparin in men with unstable coronary artery disease. Lancet 1990;336:827–830.
139. Antman EM, Anbe DT, Armstrong PW, et al. ACC/AHA guidelines for the management of patients with ST-elevation myocardial infarction: a report of the American College of Cardiology/American Heart Association task force on practice guidelines (Committee to Revise the 1999 Guidelines for the Management of Patients with Acute Myocardial Infarction). Bethesda, MD: American College of Cardiology Foundation and the American Heart Association, Inc, 2004. Available at www.acc.org/clinical/guidelines/stemi/index.pdf.
140. Antman EM. The search for replacements for unfractionated heparin. Circulation 2001;103:2310–2314.
141. Goodman SG, Fitchett D, Armstrong PW, et al; Integrilin and Enoxaparin Randomized Assessment of Acute Coronary Syndrome Treatment (INTERACT) Trial Investigators. Randomized evaluation of the safety and efficacy of enoxaparin versus unfractionated heparin in high-risk patients with non-ST-segment elevation acute coronary syndromes receiving the glycoprotein IIb/IIIa inhibitor eptifibatide. Circulation 2003;107:238–244.

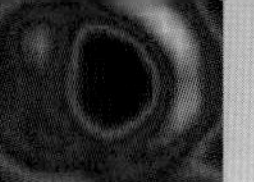

142. Blazing MA, de Lemos JA, White HD, et al; A to Z Investigators. Safety and efficacy of enoxaparin vs unfractionated heparin in patients with non-ST-segment elevation acute coronary syndromes who receive tirofiban and aspirin: a randomized controlled trial. JAMA 2004;292:55–64.
143. Ferguson JJ, Califf RM, Antman EM, et al; SYNERGY Trial Investigators. Enoxaparin vs unfractionated heparin in high-risk patients with non-ST-segment elevation acute coronary syndromes managed with an intended early invasive strategy: primary results of the SYNERGY randomized trial. JAMA 2004;292:45–54.
144. The Global Use of Strategies to Open Occluded Coronary Arteries (GUSTO) IIb investigators. A comparison of recombinant hirudin with heparin for the treatment of acute coronary syndromes. N Engl J Med 1996;335:775–782.
145. Organisation to Assess Strategies for Ischemic Syndromes (OASIS-2) Investigators. Effects of recombinant hirudin (lepirudin) compared with heparin on death, myocardial infarction, refractory angina, and revascularisation procedures in patients with acute myocardial ischaemia without ST elevation: a randomised trial. Lancet 1999;353:429–438.
146. Lincoff AM, Bittl JA, Harrington RA, et al; REPLACE-2 Investigators. Bivalirudin and provisional glycoprotein IIb/IIIa blockade compared with heparin and planned glycoprotein IIb/IIIa blockade during percutaneous coronary intervention: REPLACE-2 randomized trial. JAMA 2003;289:853–863.
147. Mehta SR. Efficacy and safety of fondaparinux compared to enoxaparin in 20,000 high risk patients with ACS without ST elevation: the OASIS 5 Michelangelo programme. Presented at ESC Congress 2005 Stockholm, 05 September 2005. Available online: http://www.escardio.org/knowledge/OnlineLearning/slides/ESC_Congress_2005/Mehta-FP1332/
148. TIMI IIIB Investigators. Effects of tissue plasminogen activator and a comparison of early invasive and conservative strategies in unstable angina and non-Q-wave myocardial infarction. Results of the TIMI IIIB trial. Thrombolysis in myocardial ischemia. Circulation 1994;89:1545–1556.
149. Boden WE, O'Rourke RA, Crawford MH, et al. Outcomes in patients with acute non-Q-wave myocardial infarction randomly assigned to an invasive as compared with a conservative management strategy. N Engl J Med 1998;338:1785–1792.
150. FRagmin and Fast Revascularization during InStability in Coronary artery disease investigators. Invasive compared with non-invasive treatment in unstable coronary-artery disease: the FRISC-II prospective randomised trial. Lancet 2000;356:9–16.
151. Cannon CP, Weintraub WS, Demopoulos LA, et al. Comparison of early invasive and conservative strategies in patients with unstable coronary syndromes treated with the glycoprotein IIb/IIIa inhibitor tirofiban. N Engl J Med 2001;344:879–887.
152. Fox KAA, Poole-Wilson PA, Henderson RA, et al; Randomized Intervention trial of unstable Angina Investigators. Interventional versus conservative treatment for patients with unstable angina or non-ST-elevation myocardial infarction: The British Heart Foundation RITA 3 randomised trial. Lancet 2002;360:743–751.
153. de Winter RJ, Windhausen F, Cornel JH, et al. Early invasive versus selectively invasive management for acute coronary syndromes. N Engl J Med 2005;353:1095–1104.
154. Newman F-J, Kastrati A, Pogatsa-Murray G, et al. Assessment of the value of cooling-off strategy (extended antithrombotic pretreatment) in patients with unstable coronary syndromes treated invasively: The Intracoronary Stenting with Antithrombotic Regiment Cooling-Off (ISAR-COOL) Trial. (Late breaking clinical trial abstract). Circulation 2003;106:2986-a.
155. Antman EM, Anhbe DT, Armstrong PW, et al. ACC/AHA guidelines for the management of patients with ST-elevation myocardial infarction–executive summary. J Am Coll Cardiol 2004;44:671–719.
156. Morrow DA, Antman EM, Giugliano RP, et al. A simple risk index for rapid initial triage of patients with ST-elevation myocardial infarction: an InTIME II substudy. Lancet 2001;358:1571–1575.
157. William DO. Treatment delayed is treatment denied. Circulation 2004;109:1806–1808.
158. Morrison LJ, Verbeek PR, McDonald AC, et al. Mortality and prehospital thrombolysis for acute myocardial infarction: a meta-analysis. JAMA 2000;283:2686–2692.
159. Morrow DA, Antman EM, Sayah A, et al. Evaluation of time saved by prehospital initiation of reteplase for ST-elevation myocardial infarction: results of the Early Retavase-Thrombolysis in Myocardial Infarction (ER-TIMI) 19 trial. J Am Coll Cardiol 2002;40:71–77.
160. Zeymer U, Tebbe U, Essen R, et al; for the ALKK-Study group. Influence of time to treatment on early infarct-related artery patency after different thrombolytic regimens. Am Heart J 1999;137:34–38.
161. Bonnefoy E, Lapostolle F, Leizorovicz A, et al. Primary angioplasty vs prehospital fibrinolysis in acute myocardial infarction: a randomised study. Lancet 2002;360:825–829.
162. Myocardial Infarction National Audit Project (MINAP). How the NHS manages heart attacks. Fourth Public Report 2005. London: Clinical Effectiveness and Evaluation Unit, Royal College of Physicians (RCP) of London, 2005. ISBN 1 86016 240 1. (see www.rcplondon.ac.uk/pubs/books/minap05/index.htm)
163. Grubel PA, Cummings CC, Bell CR, et al. Onset and extent of platelet inhibition by clopidogrel loading in patients undergoing elective coronary stenting: the Plavix Reduction of New Thrombus Occurrence (PRONTO) trial. Am Heart J 2003;145:239–247.
164. Sabatine MS, Cannon CP, Gibson CM, et al; CLARITY-TIMI 28 Investigators. Addition of clopidogrel to aspirin and fibrinolytic therapy for myocardial infarction with ST-segment elevation. N Engl J Med 2005;352:1179–1189.
165. Collins R; for the COMMIT/CCS-2 Trial Investigators. The COMMIT/CCS-2 Trial. Presented at the American College of Cardiology 54th Annual Scientific Session Late Breaking Trial III 09/03/05.
166. Gruppo Italiano per lo Studio dela Sopravvivenza nel'Infarto Miocardico. GISSI-3: effects of lisinopril and transdermal glyceryl trinitrate singly and together on 6-week mortality and ventricular function after acute myocardial infarction. Lancet 1994;343:1115–1122.
167. ISIS-4 Collaborative Group. ISIS-4: a randomized factorial trial assessing early oral captopril, oral mononitrate, and intravenous magnesium sulfate in 58050 patients with suspected acute myocardial infarction. Lancet 1995;345:669–685.
168. Schwartz GG, Olsson AG, Ezekowitz MD, et al; Myocardial Ischemia Reduction with Aggressive Cholesterol Lowering (MIRACL) Study Investigators. Effects of atorvastatin on early recurrent ischemic events in acute coronary syndromes: the MIRACL study: a randomized controlled trial. JAMA 2001;285:1711–1718.
169. Nissen SE, Tuzcu EM, Schoenhagen P, et al. Effect of intensive compared with moderate lipid-lowering therapy on progression of coronary atherosclerosis: a randomized controlled trial. JAMA 2004;291:1071–1080.
170. de Lemos JA, Blazing MA, Wiviott SD, et al; A to Z Investigators. Early intensive versus a delayed conservative simvastatin strategy in patients with acute coronary syndromes: phase Z of the A to Z trial. JAMA 2004;292:1307–1316.
171. Nissen SE. High-dose statins in acute coronary syndromes: not just lipid levels. JAMA 2004;292:1365–1367.
172. Olsson AG, Schwartz GG, Szarek M, et al. High-density lipoprotein, but not low-density lipoprotein cholesterol levels influence short-term prognosis after acute coronary syndrome: results from the MIRACL trial. Eur Heart J 2005;26:890–896.
173. Lefer AM, Campbell B, Shin YK, et al. Simvastatin preserves the ischemic-reperfused myocardium in normocholesterolemic rat hearts. Circulation 1999;100:178–184.

174. Spencer FA, Allegrone J, Goldberg RJ, et al; GRACE Investigators. Association of statin therapy with outcomes of acute coronary syndromes: the GRACE study. Ann Intern Med 2004;140:857–866.
175. Anderson JL, Karagounis LA, Califf RM. Meta-analysis of five reported studies on the relation of early patency grades with mortality and outcomes after myocardial infarction. Am J Cardiol 1996;78:1.
176. Ito H, Tomooka T, Sakai N, et al. Lack of myocardial perfusion immediately after successful thrombolysis, a predictor of poor recovery of left ventricular function in anterior myocardial infarction. Circulation 1992;85:1699–1705.
177. Juliard JM, Feldman LJ, Golmard JL, et al. Relation of mortality or primary angioplasty during acute myocardial infarction to door-to-Thrombolysis in Myocardial Infarction (TIMI) time. Am J Cardiol 2003;91:1401–1405.
178. De Luca G, Suryapranata H, Ottervanger JP, et al. Time delay to treatment and mortality in primary angioplasty for acute myocardial infarction: every minute of delay counts. Circulation 2004;109:1223–1225.
179. Boersma E, Maas ACP, Deckers JW, Simoons ML. Early thrombolytic treatment in acute myocardial infarction: reappraisal of the golden hour. Lancet 1996;348:771–775.
180. Keeley EC, Boura JA, Grines CL. Primary angioplasty vs intravenous thrombolytic therapy for acute myocardial infarction: a quantitative review of 23 randomised trials. Lancet 2003;361:13–20.
181. Wilson SH, Bell MR, Rihal CS, et al. Infarct artery reocclusion post primary angioplasty, stent placement, and thrombolytic therapy for acute myocardial infarction. Am Heart J 2001;141:704–710.
182. Berger PB, Ellis SG, Holmes DR Jr, et al. Relationship between delay in performing direct coronary angioplasty and early clinical outcome in patients with acute myocardial infarction: results from the GUSTO-IIb trial. Circulation 1999;100:14–20.
183. Horie H, Takahashi M, Minai K, et al. Long-term benefit of late reperfusion from acute anterior myocardial infarction with percutaneous transluminal coronary angioplasty. Circulation 1998;98:2377–2382.
184. De Luca G, Ernst N, Zijlstra F, et al. Preprocedural TIMI flow and mortality in patients with acute myocardial infarction treated by primary angioplasty. J Am Coll Cardiol 2004;43:1363–1367.
185. SPEED Group. Trial of abciximab with and without low-dose reteplase for acute myocardial infarction. Strategies for patency enhancement in the emergency department (SPEED) group. Circulation 2000;101:2788–2794.
186. Antman EM, Giuglisno RP, Gibson MC, et al. Abciximab facilitates the rate and extent of thrombolysis: results of the Thrombolysis in Myocardial Infarction (TIMI) 14 trial. Circulation 1999;99:2720–2732.
187. Gersh BJ, Stone GW, White HD, and Holmes DR. Pharmacological facilitation of primary percutaneous coronary intervention for acute myocardial infarction. JAMA 2005;293:979–986.
188. Fibrinolytic Therapy Trialists Collaborative Group. Indications for fibrinolytic therapy in suspected acute myocardial infarction: collaborative overview of early mortality and major morbidity results from all randomized trials of more than 1000 patients. Lancet 1994;343:311–322.
189. Hermentin P, Cuesta-Linker T, Weisse J, et al. Comparative analysis of the activity and content of different streptokinase preparations. Eur Heart J 2005;26:933–940.
190. The GUSTO investigators. An international trial comparing four thrombolytic strategies for acute myocardial infarction. N Engl J Med 1993;329:673–682.
191. The GUSTO Angiographic Investigators. The effects of tissue plasminogen activator, streptokinase, or both on coronary-artery patency, ventricular function, and survival after acute myocardial infarction. N Engl J Med 1993;329:1615–1622.
192. Bode C, Smalling RW, Berg G, et al. Randomized comparison of coronary thrombolysis achieved with double-bolus reteplase (recombinant plasminogen activator) and front-loaded, accelerated alteplase (recombinant tissue plasminogen activator) in patients with acute myocardial infarction. The RAPID II Investigators. Circulation 1996;94:891–898.
193. The Global Use of Strategies to Open Occluded Coronary Arteries (GUSTO) III Investigators. A comparison of reteplase with alteplase for acute myocardial infarction. N Engl J Med 1997;337:1118–1123.
194. Van der Werf FJ. The ideal fibrinolytic: can drug design improve clinical results? Eur Heart J 1999;20:1452–1458.
195. Cannon CP, Gibson CM, McCabe CH, et al. TNK-tissue plasminogen activator compared with front-loaded alteplase in acute myocardial infarction: results of the TIMI 10B trial. Thrombolysis in Myocardial Infarction (TIMI) 10B Investigators. Circulation 1998;98:2805–2814.
196. ASSENT-Investigators. Single-bolus tenecteplase compared with front-loaded alteplase in acute myocardial infarction: the ASSENT-2 double-blind randomized trial. Lancet 1999;354:716–722.
197. The Assessment of the Safety and Efficacy of a New Thrombolytic Regimen (ASSENT)-3 Investigators. Efficacy and safety of tenecteplase in combination with enoxaparin, abciximab, or unfractionated heparin: the ASSENT-3 randomised trial in acute myocardial infarction. Lancet 2001:358:605–613.
198. Granger CB, White HD, Bates ER, et al. A pooled analysis of coronary patency and left ventricular function after intravenous thrombolysis for acute myocardial infarction. Am J Cardiol 1994;74:1220–1228.
199. Menon V, Harrington RA, Hochman JS, et al. Thrombolysis and adjunctive therapy in acute myocardial infarction: the Seventh ACCP Conference on Antithrombotic and Thrombolytic Therapy. Chest 2004;126(3 Suppl):549S–575S.
200. Topol EJ. Reperfusion therapy for acute myocardial infarction with fibrinolytic therapy or combination reduced fibrinolytic therapy and platelet glycoprotein IIb/IIIa inhibition: the GUSTO V randomised trial. Lancet 2001;357:1905–1914.
201. De Luca G, Suryapranata H, Stone GW, et al. Abciximab as adjunctive therapy to reperfusion in acute ST-segment elevation myocardial infarction: a meta-analysis of randomized trials. JAMA 2005;293:1759–1765.
202. Lee DP, Herity NA, Hiatt BL, et al. Adjunctive platelet glycoprotein IIb/IIIa receptor inhibition with tirofiban before primary angioplasty improves angiographic outcomes: results of the TIrofiban Given in the Emergency Room before Primary Angioplasty (TIGER-PA) pilot trial. Circulation 2003;107:1497–1501.
203. Zeymer U, Zahn R, Schiele R, et al. Early eptifibatide improves TIMI 3 patency before primary percutaneous coronary intervention for acute ST elevation myocardial infarction: results of the randomized integrilin in acute myocardial infarction (INTAMI) pilot trial. Eur Heart J 2005. Available at: http://www.eurheartj.oxfordjournals.org/cgi/content/abstract/ehi293v1.
204. Savonitto S, Armstrong PW, Lincoff AM, et al; GUSTO V Investigators. Risk of intracranial haemorrhage with combined fibrinolytic and glycoprotein IIb/IIIa inhibitor therapy in acute myocardial infarction: dichotomous response as a function of age in the GUSTO V trial. Eur Heart J 2003;24:1807–1814.
205. Montalescot G, Barragan P, Wittenberg O, et al; ADMIRAL Investigators. Platelet glycoprotein IIb/IIIa inhibition with coronary stenting for acute myocardial infarction. N Engl J Med 2001;344:1895–1903.
206. Gurwirtz JH, Gore JM, Goldberg RJ, et al. Risk for intracranial hemorrhage after tissue plasminogen activator treatment for acute myocardial infarction. Ann Intern Med 1998;129:597–604.
207. Van der Werf F, Barron HV, Armstrong PW, et al; ASSENT-2 Investigators. Incidence and predictors of bleeding events after fibrinolytic therapy with fibrin-specific agents: a comparison of TNK-tPA and rt-PA. Eur Heart J 2001;22:2253–2261.
208. Andersen HR, Nielsen TT, Rasmussen K, et al. A comparison of coronary angioplasty with fibrinolytic therapy in acute myocardial infarction. N Engl J Med 2003;349:733–742.

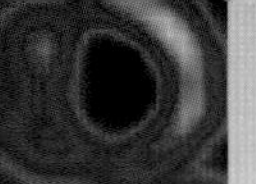

209. Van de Werf F, Gore JM, Avezum A, et al. Access to catheterisation facilities in patients admitted with acute coronary syndrome: multinational registry study. BMJ 2005;330:441–444.
210. Dalby M, Bouzamondo A, Lechat P, Montalescot G. Transfer for primary angioplasty versus immediate thrombolysis in acute myocardial infarction. A meta-analysis. Circulation 2003:108:1809–1814.
211. Smith D, Channer KS. For and against. Primary angioplasty should be first line treatment for acute myocardial infarction. BMJ 2004:328:1254–1257.
212. Grines CL, Cox DA, Stone GW, et al; Stent Primary Angioplasty in Myocardial Infarction Study Group. Coronary angioplasty with and without stent implantation for acute myocardial infarction. N Engl J Med 1999;341:1949–1956.
213. Maillard L, Hamon M, Khalife K, et al; STENTIM-2 investigators. A comparison of systematic stenting and conventional balloon angioplasty during primary percutaneous transluminal coronary angioplasty for acute myocardial infarction. J Am Coll Cardiol 2000;35:1729–1736.
214. Moses JW, Leon MB, Popma JJ, et al. Sirolimus-eluting stents versus standard stents in patients with stenosis in a native coronary artery. N Engl J Med 2003;349:1315–1323.
215. Stone GW. TAXUS-IV: clinical results of the pivotal prospective, multicenter, randomised trial of the polymer-based paclitaxel-eluting stent in patients with de novo lesions. Presented at Transcatheter Cardiovascular Theraputics 2003, Washington, DC, September 2003.
216. Lemos PA, Saia F, Hofma SH, et al. Short- and long-term clinical benefit of sirolimus-eluting stents compared to conventional bare metal stents for patients with acute myocardial infarction. J Am Coll Cardiol 2004;43:704–708.
217. The TIMI study group. The thrombolysis in myocardial infarction (TIMI) trial. N Engl J Med 1985;31:932–936.
218. Davies CH, Ormerod OJ. Failed thrombolysis. Lancet 1998;351:1191–1196.
219. Goldman LE, Eisenberg MJ. Identification and management of patients with failed thrombolysis after acute myocardial infarction. Ann Intern Med 2000;132:556–565.
220. Schomig A, Ndrepepa G, Mehilli J, et al. A randomized trial of coronary stenting versus balloon angioplasty as a rescue intervention after failed thrombolysis in patients with acute myocardial infarction. J Am Coll Cardiol 2004;14:2073–2079.
221. Gershlick A. Rescue angioplasty versus conservative treatment or repeat thrombolysis (REACT). Presented at: Annual Scientific Session of the American Heart Association, New Orleans, Louisiana, November 2004.
222. Johanson P, Jernberg T, Gunnarsson G, et al. Prognostic value of ST-segment resolution – when and what to measure. Eur Heart J 2003;24:337–345.
223. Ross AM, Gibons RJ, Stone GW, et al. A randomized, double-blinded, placebo-controlled multicenter trial of adenosine as an adjunct to reperfusion in the treatment of acute myocardial infarction (AMISTAD II). J Am Coll Cardiol 2005;45:1775–1780.
224. Sugimoto K, Ito H, Iwakura K, et al. IV nicorandil in conjunction with coronary reperfusion is associated with better clinical and functional outcome in patients with AMI. Circ J 2003;67:295–300.
225. Ikeda N, Yasu T, Kubo N, et al. Nicorandil vs. isosorbide dinitrate as an adjunct to direct balloon angioplasty in acute myocardial infarction. Heart 2004;90:181–185.
226. Stone G, Brodie BR, Griffin JJ, et al. Role of cardiac surgery in the hospital phase management of patients treated with primary angioplasty for acute myocardial infarction. Am J Cardiol 2000;85:1292–1296.
227. Fibrinolysis Therapy Trialists (FTT) Collaborative Group. Indications for fibrinolytic therapy in suspected acute myocardial infarction: collaborative overview of early mortality and major morbidity results from all randomized trials of more than 1000 patients. Lancet 1994;343:311–322.
228. Mehta RH, Granger CB, Alexander KP, et al. Reperfusion strategies for acute myocardial infarction in the elderly: benefits and risks. J Am Coll Cardiol 2005;45:471–478.
229. Hochman JS, Sleeper LA, Webb JG, et al; Should We Emergently Revascularize Occluded Arteries for Cardiogenic Shock (SHOCK) Investigators. Early revascularization in acute myocardial infarction complicated by cardiogenic shock. N Engl J Med 1999;341:625–634.
230. Dzavik V, Sleeper LA, Cocke TP, et al; SHOCK investigators. Early revascularization is associated with improved survival in elderly patients with acute myocardial infarction complicated by shock: a report of the SHOCK trial registry. Eur Heart J 2003;24:828–837.
231. Centers for Disease Control and Prevention (CDC). Trends in ageing–United States and worldwide. MMWR Morb Mortal Wkly Rep 2003;52:101–104, 106.
232. Lampe FC, Morris RW, Walker M, et al. Trends in rates of different forms of diagnosed coronary heart disease, 1978–2000: prospective population based study of British men. BMJ 2005;330:1046–1049.
233. Bulpitt CJ. Secondary prevention of coronary heart disease in the elderly. Heart 2005;91:396–400.
234. Spencer FA, Goldberg RJ, Frederick PD, et al. Age and the utilisation of cardiac catheterisation following uncomplicated first acute myocardial infarction treated with thrombolytic therapy (the Second National Registry of Myocardial Infarction NRMI-2). Am J Cardiol 2001;88:107–111.
235. Zieman S, Schulman S, Fleg J. Ischaemic heart disease. Ageing, Heart Disease and its Management 2003:249–273.
236. Kaufman D, Kelly JP, Rosenberg L, et al. Recent patterns of medication use in the ambulatory adult population of the United States. The Sloane survey. JAMA 2002;287:337.
237. Moore JG, Bjorkman DJ, Mitchell MD, Avots-Avontins A. Age does not influence acute aspirin-induced gastric mucosal damage. Gastroenterology 1991;100:1626–1629.
238. Buresly K, Eisenberg MJ, Zhang X, Pilote L. Bleeding complications associated with combinations of aspirin, thienopyridine derivatives, and warfarin in elderly patients following acute myocardial infarction. Arch Intern Med 2005;165:784–789.
239. Gottlieb SS, McCarter RJ, Vogel RA. Effect of beta blockade on mortality among high-risk and low-risk patients after myocardial infarction. N Engl J Med 1998;339:489–497.
240. Chen J, Radford MJ, Wang Y, et al. Effectiveness of beta blocker therapy after myocardial infarction in elderly patients with chronic obstructive pulmonary disease or asthma. J Am Coll Cardiol 2001;37:1950–1956.
241. ACE inhibitor myocardial infarction collaborative group. Indications for ACE inhibitors in the early treatment of acute myocardial infarction. Circulation 1998;97:2202–2212.
242. Scandinavian Simvastatin Survival Study. Randomised trial of cholesterol lowering in 4444 patients with coronary heart disease. The Scandinavian Simvastatin Survival Study (4S). Lancet 1994;344:1383–1389.
243. Sacks FM, Pfeffer MA, Moye LA, et al. The effect of pravastatin on coronary events after myocardial infarction in patients with average cholesterol levels. N Engl J Med 1996;335:1001–1009.
244. Antman E, Cohen M, Radley D, et al. Assessment of the treatment effect of enoxaparin for unstable angina/non Q wave myocardial infarction. TIMI II B-ESSENCE meta-analysis. Circulation 1999;100:1602–1608.
245. Menon V, Berkowitz SD, Antman EM, et al. New heparin dosing recommendations for patients with acute coronary syndromes. Am J Med 2001;110:641–650.

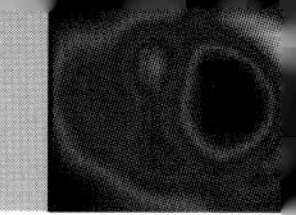

246. Berger A. Thrombolysis in elderly patients with acute myocardial infarction. Am J Geriatr Cardiol 2003;12:251–256.
247. White HD, Barbash GI, Califf RM, et al. Age and outcomes with contemporary thrombolytic therapy. Results from the GUSTO-1 trial. Circulation 1996;94:1826–1833.
248. Thiemann DR, Coresh J, Schulman SP, et al. Lack of benefit of intravenous thrombolysis in patients with myocardial infarction who are older than 75. Circulation 2000;101:2239–2246.
249. Soumerai SB, McLaughlin TJ, Ross-Degnan D, et al. Effectiveness of thrombolytic therapy for acute myocardial infarction in the elderly: cause for concern in the old-old. Arch Intern Med 2002;162:561–568.
250. Berger AK, Radford MJ, Wang Y, et al. Thrombolytic therapy in older patients. J Am Coll Cardiol 2000;36:366–374.
251. Gitt AK, Zahn R, Wienberger H, et al. Thrombolysis for acute myocardial infarction in patients older than 75 years: lack of benefit for hospital mortality but improvement of long-term mortality: results of the MITRA- and MIR- registries. J Am Coll Cardiol 2001;37(Suppl A):1A–648A. Abstract No. 1086-93.
252. Berger AK, Schulman KA, Gersh BJ, et al. Primary coronary angioplasty vs thrombolysis for the management of acute myocardial infarction in elderly patients. JAMA 1999;282:341–348.
253. Mehta R, Sadiq I, Goldberg R, et al. Effectiveness of primary percutaneous coronary intervention compared with that of thrombolytic therapy in elderly patients with acute myocardial infarction. Am Heart J 2004;147:253–259.
254. DeGeare VS, Stone GW, Grines L, et al. Angiographic and clinical characteristics associated with increased in-hospital mortality in elderly patients with acute myocardial infarction undergoing percutaneous intervention (a pooled analysis of the primary angioplasty in myocardial infarction trials). Am J Cardiol 2000;86:30–34.
255. Hochman JS, Buller CE, Sleeper LA. Cardiogenic shock complicating acute myocardial infarction – aetiologies, management and outcome; overall findings of the SHOCK trial registry. J Am Coll Cardiol 2000;36:1063–1070.
256. Peterson ED, Cowper PA, Jollis JG, et al. Outcomes of coronary artery bypass graft surgery in 24461 patients aged 80yrs or older. Circulation 1995;92(9 Suppl):II85–91.
257. Roach GW, Kanchuger M, Mangano CM. Adverse cerebral outcomes after coronary bypass surgery. N Engl J Med 1996;335:1857–1863.
258. Newman MF, Kirchner JL, Phillips-Bute B. Longitudinal assessment of neurocognitive function after coronary-artery bypass surgery. N Engl J Med 2001;344:395–402.
259. Peterson E, Alexander K, Malenka D, et al. Multicentre experience in revascularisation of very elderly patients. Am Heart J 2004;148:486–492.
260. Chaturvedi N. Ethnic differences in cardiovascular disease. Heart 2003;89:681–686.
261. Mensah GA, Mokdad AH, Ford ES, et al. State of disparities in cardiovascular health in the United States. Circulation 2005;111:1233–1241.
262. Yancy CW, Benjamin EJ, Fabunmi RP, Bonow RO. Discovering the full spectrum of cardiovascular disease. Minority Health Summit 2003. Circulation 2005;111:1339–1349.
263. Sonel AF, Good CB, Mulgand J, et al. Racial variations in treatment and outcomes of black and white patients with high-risk non-ST-elevation acute coronary syndromes. Circulation 2005;111:1225–1232.
264. Sabatine MS, Blake GJ, Drazner MH, et al. Influence of race on death and ischemic complications in patients with non-ST-elevation acute coronary syndromes despite modern, protocol-guided treatment. Circulation 2005;111:1217–1224.
265. Kaul P, Lytle BL, Spertus JA, et al. Influence of racial disparities in procedure use on functional status outcomes among patients with coronary artery disease. Circulation 2005;111:1284–1290.
266. Kuppuswamy VC, Gupta S. Excess coronary heart disease in South Asians in the United Kingdom. BMJ 2005;330:1223–1224.
267. Patel H, Rosengren A, Ekman I, et al. Symptoms in acute coronary syndromes: does sex make a difference? Am Heart J 2004;148:27–33.
268. Morise AP, Diamond GA. Comparison of the sensitivity and specificity of exercise electrocardiography in biased and unbiased populations of men and women. Am Heart J 1995;130:741–747.
269. Wiviott SD, Cannon CP, Morrow DA, et al. Differential expression of cardiac biomarkers by gender in patients with unstable angina/non-ST-elevation myocardial infarction: a TACTICS-TIMI 18 (Treat Angina with Aggrastat and determine Cost of Therapy with an Invasive or Conservative Strategy-Thrombolysis In Myocardial Infarction 18) substudy. Circulation 2004;109:580–586.
270. Blomkalns AL, Chen AY, Hochman JS, et al. Gender disparities in the diagnosis and treatment of non-ST-segment elevation acute coronary syndromes: large-scale observations from the CRUSADE (Can Rapid Risk Stratification of Unstable Angina Patients Suppress Adverse Outcomes With Early Implementation of the American College of Cardiology/American Heart Association Guidelines) National Quality Improvement Initiative. J Am Coll Cardiol 2005;45:832–837.
271. Wenger NK. Coronary heart disease: the female heart is vulnerable. Prog Cardiovasc Dis 2003;46:199–229.
272. Mak KH, Kark JD, Chia KS, et al. Ethnic variations in female vulnerability after an acute myocardial infarction. Heart 2004;90:621–626.
273. Lansky AJ. Outcomes of percutaneous and surgical revascularization in women. Prog Cardiovasc Dis 2004;46:305–319.
274. Lanza GA. Ethnic variations in acute coronary syndromes. Heart 2005;90:595–597.
275. Lane DA, Lip GYH, Beevers DG. Ethnic differences in cardiovascular and all-cause mortality in Birmingham, England: The Birmingham Factory Screening Project. J Hypertens 2005;23:1347–1353.
276. Yusuf S, Hawken S, Ôunpuu S, et al. Effect of potentially modifiable risk factors associated with myocardial infarction in 52 countries (the INTERHEART study): case control study. Lancet 2004;364:937–952. Available at: http://image.thelancet.com/extras/04art8001web.pdf.
277. Unal B, Critchley JA, Capewell S. Explaining the decline in coronary heart disease mortality in England and Wales between 1981 and 2000. Circulation 2004;109:1101–1107.
278. Joseph AM, Fu SS. Smoking cessation for patients with cardiovascular disease. What is the best approach? Am J CV Drugs 2003;3(5):339–349.
279. Twardella D, Küpper-Nybelen J, Rothenbacher D, et al. Short-term benefit of smoking cessation in patients with coronary artery disease: estimates based on self-reported smoking data and serum cotinine measurements. Eur Heart J 2004;25:2101–2108.
280. Trichopoulou A, Orfanos P, Norat T, et al. Modified Mediterranean diet and survival: EPIC-elderly perspective cohort study. BMJ 2005;330:991–995.
281. Grundy SM, Cleeman JI, Merz CNB, et al. Implications of recent clinical trials for the National Cholesterol Education Program Adult Treatment Panel III Guidelines. Circulation 2004;110:227–239.
282. Shepherd J, Cobbe SM, Ford I, et al. Prevention of coronary heart disease with pravastatin in men with hypercholesterolaemia. West of Scotland Coronary Prevention Study Group (WOSCOPS). N Engl J Med 1995;16;333(20):1301–1307.

283. Downs JR, Clearfield M, Weis S, et al. Primary prevention of acute coronary events with lovastatin in men and women with average cholesterol levels: results of Air Force/Texas Coronary Atherosclerosis Prevention Study (AFCAPS/TexCAPS). JAMA 1998;279:1615–1622.
284. Sever PS, Dahlof B, Poulter NR, et al. Prevention of coronary and stroke events with atorvastatin in hypertensive patients who have average or lower than average cholesterol concentrations, in the Anglo-Scandinavian Cardiac Outcomes Trial – Lipid Lowering Arm (ASCOT-LLA): a multicentre randomised controlled trial. Lancet 2003;361:1149–1158.
285. O'Keefe JH, Cordain L, Harris WH, et al. Optimal low-density lipoprotein is 50 to 70 mg/dl. Lower is better and physiologically normal. J Am Coll Cardiol 2004;43:2142–2146.
286. Scandinavian Simvastatin Survival Study Group. Randomised trial of cholesterol lowering in 4444 patients with coronary heart disease: the Scandinavian Simvastatin Study (4S). Lancet 1994;344:1383–1389.
287. The Long-Term Intervention with Pravastatin in Ischaemic Disease (LIPID) Study Group. Prevention of cardiovascular events and deaths with pravastatin in patients with coronary heart disease and a broad range of initial cholesterol levels. N Engl J Med 1998;339:1349–1357.
288. Heart Protection Study Collaborative Group. MRC/BHF Heart Protection Study of cholesterol lowering with simvastatin in 20 536 high-risk individuals: a randomised placebo-controlled trial. Lancet 2002;360:7–22.
289. Ridker PM, Cannon CP, Morrow D, et al. C-reactive protein levels and outcomes after statin therapy. N Engl J Med 2005;352:20–28.
290. Nissen SE, Tuzcu EM, Schoenhagen P, et al. Statin therapy, LDL cholesterol, C-reactive protein, and coronary artery disease. N Engl J Med 2005;352:29–38.
291. Cholesterol Treatment Trialists' (CCT) Collaborators. Efficacy and safety of cholesterol-lowering treatment: prospective meta-analysis of data from 90 056 participants in 14 randomised trials of statins. Lancet 2005. Published online September 27 2005 DOI:10.1016/So140-6736(05)67394-1. www.thelancet.com.
292. La Rosa JC, Grundy SM, Waters DD, et al. Intensive lipid lowering with atorvastatin in patients with coronary artery disease. N Engl J Med 2005;352:1425–1435.
293. Superko HR. Beyond LDL cholesterol reduction. Circulation 1996;94:2351–2354.
294. De Backer G, Ambrosioni E, Borch-Johnsen K, et al. European guidelines on cardiovascular disease. Third Joint Task Force of European and other Societies on Cardiovascular Disease Prevention in Clinical Practice. Eur J Cardiovasc Prevention Rehab 2003;10(Suppl 1):S1–S78.
295. Ballantyne CM. Changing lipid-lowering guidelines: whom to treat and how low to go. Eur Heart J 2005;7(Suppl A):A12–A19.
296. Shepherd J. Combined lipid lowering drug therapy for the effective treatment of hypercholesterolaemia. Eur Heart J 2003;24:685–689.
297. Gagne C, Bays HE, Weiss SR, et al. Efficacy and safety of ezetimibe added to ongoing statin therapy for treatment of patients with primary hypercholesterolemia. Am J Cardiol 2002;90:1084–1091.
298. Gotto AM, et al. ILIB Lipid Handbook for Clinical Practice. Dyslipidemia and Coronary Heart Disease. 3rd edition. New York: International Lipid Information Bureau, 2003.
299. Betteridge DJ, Morrell JM. Clinicians Guide to Lipids and Coronary Heart Disease. 2nd edition. London: Arnold Publications, 2003.
300. Toth PP. High-density lipoprotein and cardiovascular risk. Circulation 2004;109:1809–1812.
301. Bloomfield Rubins H, Robins SJ, Collins D, et al. Gemfibrozil for the secondary prevention of coronary heart disease in men with low levels of high-density lipoprotein cholesterol. N Engl J Med 1999;341:410–418.
302. Canner PL, Furberg CD, Terrin ML, McGovern ME. Benefits of niacin by glycemic status in patients with healed myocardial infarction (from the Coronary Drug Project). Am J Cardiol 2005;95:254–257.
303. Marchioli R, Barzi F, Bomba E, et al. Early protection against sudden death by n-3 polyunsaturated fatty acids after myocardial infarction: time-course analysis of results of the Gruppo Italiano per lo Studio della Sopravvivenza nell'Infarto Miocardico (GISSI)-Prevenzione. Circulation 2002;105:1874–1875.
304. Kannel WB. Blood pressure as a cardiovascular risk factor. JAMA 1996;275:1571–1576.
305. Sever P. Anglo-Scandinavian Cardiac Outcomes Trial (ASCOT): a randomized, controlled trial of the prevention of CHD and other vascular events by BP and cholesterol lowering in a factorial study design. Presentation, 54th Annual Scientific Session, American College of Cardiology, Orlando, Fl, USA, 2005.
306. The Heart Outcomes Prevention Evaluation Study Investigators. Effects of an angiotensin-converting enzyme inhibitor, ramipril, on cardiovascular events in high-risk patients. N Engl J Med 2000;342:145–153.
307. The EURopean trial On reduction of cardiac events with Perindopril in stable coronary Artery disease Investigators. Efficacy of perindopril in reduction of cardiovascular events among patients with stable coronary artery disease: randomised, double-blind, placebo-controlled, multicentre trial (the EUROPA study). Lancet 2003;362:782–788.
308. Braunwald E, Domanski MJ, Fowler SE, et al. Angiotensin-converting-enzyme inhibition in stable coronary artery disease. The PEACE trial investigators. N Engl J Med 2004;351:2058–2117.
309. Pfeffer MA, McMurray JJV, Velazquez EJ, et al. Valsartan, captopril, or both in myocardial infarction complicated by heart failure, left ventricular dysfunction, or both. N Engl J Med 2003;349:1893–1906.
310. British Heart Foundation. European cardiovascular disease statistics. London: British Heart Foundation, 2005. Available at: www.heartstats.org.
311. Van Gaal LF, Rissanen AM, Scheen A, et al. Effects of the cannabinoid-1 receptor blocker rimonabant on weight reduction and cardiovascular risk factors in overweight patients: 1-year experience from the RIO-Europe study. Lancet 2005;365:1389–1397.
312. Official PROactive results website www.proactive-results.com/index.htm (accessed 15 September 2005).
313. Freemantle N. How well does the evidence on pioglitazone back up researchers' claims for a reduction in macrovascular events? BMJ 2005;331:836–838.
314. Leon AS, Franklin BA, Costa F, et al. Cardiac rehabilitation and secondary prevention of coronary heart disease. Circulation 2005;111:369–376.
315. Yusuf S. Two decades of progress in preventing vascular disease. Lancet 2002;360:2–3.
316. Wald NJ, Law MR. A strategy to reduce cardiovascular disease by more than 80%. BMJ 2003;326:1419.
317. Lesperance F, Frasure-Smith N, Juneau M, Théroux P. Depression at 1-year prognosis in unstable angina. Arch Intern Med 2000;160:1354–1360.
318. Saikku P, Leinonen M, Mattila K, et al. Serological evidence of an association of a novel Chlamydia, TWAR, with chronic coronary heart disease and acute myocardial infarction. Lancet 1988;2:983–986.

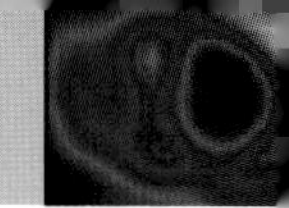

319. Maass M, Bartels C, Engel PM, et al. Endovascular presence of viable Chlamydia pneumoniae is a common phenomenon in coronary artery disease. J Am Coll Cardiol 1998;31:827–832.
320. Kuo C, Campbell LA. Detection of Chlamydia pneumoniae in arterial tissues. J Infect Dis 2000;181(Suppl 3):S432–S436.
321. Fong IW, Chiu B, Viira E, et al. De novo induction of atherosclerosis by Chlamydia pneumoniae in a rabbit model. Infect Immun 1999;67:6048–6055.
322. Gupta S, Leatham EW, Carrington D, et al. Elevated Chlamydia pneumoniae antibodies, cardiovascular events, and azithromycin in male survivors of myocardial infarction. Circulation 1997;96:404–407.
323. Gurfinkel E, Bozovich G, Daroca A, et al; ROXIS Study Group. Randomised trial of roxithromycin in non-Q-wave coronary syndromes: ROXIS Pilot Study. Lancet 1997;350:404–407.
324. Muhlestein JB, Anderson JL, Carlquist JF, et al. Randomized secondary prevention trial of azithromycin in patients with coronary artery disease: primary clinical results of the ACADEMIC study. Circulation 2000;102:1755–1760.
325. Stone AF, Mendall MA, Kaski JC, et al. Effect of treatment for Chlamydia pneumoniae and Helicobacter pylori on markers of inflammation and cardiac events in patients with acute coronary syndromes: South Thames trial of antibiotics in myocardial infarction and unstable angina (STAMINA). Circulation 2002;106:1219–1223.
326. Burkhardt U, Zahn R, Hoffler U. Antibody levels against Chlamydia pneumoniae and outcome of roxithromycin therapy in patients with acute myocardial infarction. Results from a sub-study of the randomised Antibiotic Therapy in Acute Myocardial Infarction (ANTIBIO) trial. Cardiology 2004;93(9):671–678.
327. Neumann F, Kastrati A, Miethke T, et al. Treatment of Chlamydia pneumoniae infection with roxithromycin and effect on neointima proliferation after coronary stent placement (ISAR-3): a randomised, double-blind, placebo-controlled trial. Lancet 2001;357:2085–2089.
328. Vammen S, Lindholt JS, Ostergaard L, et al. Randomized double blind controlled trial of roxithromycin for prevention of abdominal aortic aneurysm expansion. Br J Surg. 2001;88:1066–1072.
329. Wiesli P, Czerwenka W, Meniconi A, et al. Roxithromycin treatment prevents progression of peripheral arterial occlusive disease in Chlamydia pneumoniae seropositive men. Circulation 2002;105:2646–2652.
330. Sander D, Winbeck K, Klingelhofer J, et al. Progression of early carotid atherosclerosis is only temporarily reduced after antibiotic treatment of Chlamydia pneumoniae seropositivity. Circulation 2004;109:1010–1015.
331. O'Connor CM, Dunne MW, Pfeffer MA, et al; investigators in the WIZARD [Weekly Intervention with Zithromax for Atherosclerosis and its Related Disorders] Study. Azithromycin for the secondary prevention of coronary heart disease events: the WIZARD study: a randomized controlled trial. JAMA 2003;290:1459–1466.
332. Grayston JT, Kronmal RA, Jackson LA, et al; ACES Investigators. Azithromycin for the secondary prevention of coronary events. N Engl J Med 2005;352:1637–1645.
333. Cercek B, Shah PK, Noc M, et al; AZACS Investigators. Effect of short-term treatment with azithromycin on recurrent ischaemic events in patients with acute coronary syndrome in the Azithromycin in Acute Coronary Syndrome (AZACS) trial: a randomised controlled trial. Lancet 2003;361:809–813.
334. Cannon CP, Braunwald E, McCabe CH, et al. The Pravastatin or Atorvastatin Evaluation and Infection Therapy (PROVE-IT). Antibiotic treatment of Chlamydia pneumoniae after acute coronary syndrome. N Engl J Med 2005;352:1646–1654.
335. Ngeh J, Gupta S. Inflammation, infection and antimicrobial therapy in coronary heart disease – where do we currently stand? Fundam Clin Pharmacol 2001;15:85–93.
336. Wells BJ, Mainous AG, Dickerson LM. Antibiotics for the secondary prevention of ischemic heart disease: a meta-analysis of randomized controlled trials. Arch Intern Med 2004;164:2156–2161.
337. Danesh J. Antibiotics in the prevention of heart attacks. Lancet 2005;365:809–811.
338. Anderson JL. Infection, antibiotics, and atherothrombosis – end of the road or new beginnings? N Engl J Med 2005;352:1706–1709.
339. Andraws R, Berger JS, Brown DL. Effects of antibiotic therapy on outcomes of patients with coronary artery disease: a meta-analysis of randomized controlled trials. JAMA 2005;293:2641–2647.

Index

Notes: As the subject of this book is acute coronary syndromes (ACS) all entries refer to this subject unless otherwise stated. Page numbers in *italics* refer to figures. Abbreviations used in the index can be found on pages 137–142.

A

B

C

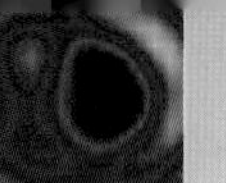

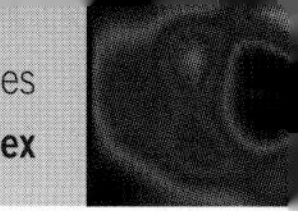

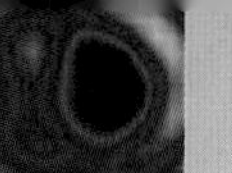

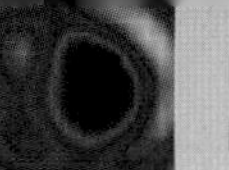

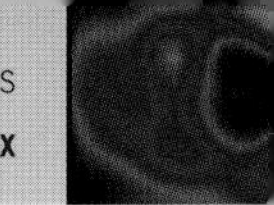

P

R

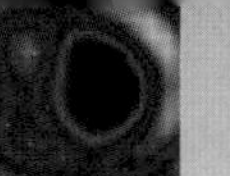

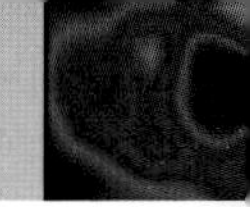